Embryolog

AN ILLUSTRATED COLOUR

Commissioning Editor: Timothy Horne
Project Editor: Lynn Watt
Project Controller: Nancy Arnott
Designer: Erik Bigland
Illustration Manager: Bruce Hogarth

Embryology

AN ILLUSTRATED COLOUR TEXT

Barry Mitchell BSc MSc PhD FIBMS FIBiol
Director, Centre for Learning Anatomical Sciences
School of Medicine, University of Southampton
Southampton, UK

Ram Sharma BSc MSc PhD
Lecturer, Centre for Learning Anatomical Sciences
School of Medicine, University of Southampton
Southampton, UK

Student advisor: M. I. Dykes

Illustrated by Robert Britton

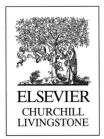

ELSEVIER
CHURCHILL
LIVINGSTONE

EDINBURGH   LONDON   NEW YORK   OXFORD   PHILADELPHIA   ST LOUIS   SYDNEY   TORONTO   2005

ELSEVIER | CHURCHILL LIVINGSTONE
An imprint of Elsevier Limited

First published 2005
Reprinted 2005, 2007

ISBN 13: 978 0443 073984
ISBN 10: 0443 073988

British Library Cataloguing in Publication Data
A catalogue record for this book is available from the British Library

Library of Congress Cataloging in Publication Data
A catalog record for this book is available from the Library of Congress

> **Notice**
> Medical knowledge is constantly changing. Standard safety precautions must be followed, but as new research and clinical experience broaden our knowledge, changes in treatment and drug therapy may become necessary or appropriate. Readers are advised to check the most current product information provided by the manufacturer of each drug to be administered to verify the recommended dose, the method and duration of administration, and contraindications. It is the responsibility of the practitioner, relying on experience and knowledge of the patient, to determine dosages and the best treatment for each individual patient. Neither the Publisher nor the authors assume any liability for any injury and/or damage to persons or property arising from this publication.

ELSEVIER your source for books,
journals and multimedia
in the health sciences
www.elsevierhealth com

Working together to grow
libraries in developing countries
www.elsevier.com | www.bookaid.org | www.sabre.org
ELSEVIER   BOOKAID International   Sabre Foundation

The
publisher's
policy is to use
**paper manufactured
from sustainable forests**

Preface

Embryology provides an understanding of the process by which the human body develops. The study of embryology is essential for understanding topographical relationships in gross anatomy, and for many congenital anomalies. Embryology is a challenging subject because of the relative speed with which changes in form occur over time. This situation is compounded by the use of two- dimensional diagrams of four-dimensional events. Furthermore, this is all set in relation to descriptive terminology, which is likely to be unfamiliar to the student.

In many undergraduate medical curricula, however, as a subject, embryology has been lost or it has been significantly reduced. The aim of this book, therefore, is to provide students with a concise, illustrated text which confines its descriptions to those which are relevant for the modern medical undergraduate and postgraduate courses, and other related disciplines. The text and accompanying illustrations explain how the embryo and fetus develop. The aim is not to provide a mechanistic explanation from the point of view of developmental biology, for which there are already many satisfactory texts available. Those requiring further detail are encouraged to consult texts that provide greater depth, either in descriptive embryology or in developmental biology.

We wish to thank Dr Sil Wallach for her helpful comments on the manuscript and also Michael Dykes for his helpful and instructive comments on the text and diagrams.

Barry Mitchell
Ram Sharma
2004

Contents

Chapter 1
How does an embryo form?

Table 1.1 **Stages of development before birth**		
Time period	**Stage**	**Main events**
1st week	Cleavage	Fertilized ovum undergoes mitosis. Formation of morula; appearance of blastocyst; blastocyst implanted
2nd to 8th week	Embryonic period	Germ layers and placenta develop. Main body systems form
9th week to birth	Fetal period	Further growth and development of organs. Locomotor system becomes functional

By definition, an embryo comprises the tissues formed once mitosis of an **ovum** (a fertilized oocyte) begins, thus even at the two-cell stage it is an embryo. These few cells multiply in number over an 8-week period into a fetus, by which time it will consist of many millions of cells. The differentiation that establishes the organ systems takes place in the first 8 weeks following fertilization (the **embryonic period**). The period of time from the end of week 8 to full term (38 weeks) is a phase of growth and enlargement (the **fetal period**). The crucial phase during which there is potential for malformation is in the first 8 weeks, and this period is when the embryo is most vulnerable to environmental agents such as viruses and other **teratogens**. Table 1.1 summarizes the major events of the prenatal stages of development. The stages of the formation of an embryo are often described in relation to weeks of development.

The stages leading up to fertilization (including gametogenesis and the histology of the uterus at the time of implantation), however, are beyond the scope of this book.

The 1st week

A fertilized ovum has a diploid number of chromosomes and once the second meiotic division has been completed, the stage of cleavage can begin. This consists of a series of rapid mitotic cell divisions in which the ovum divides over a period of about 3 days resulting in the so-called 16-cell-stage embryo (Figs 1.1, 1.2A). Each cell is known as a **blastomere**. After each cleavage division, whilst the number of cells increases, the size of each cell diminishes. The solid sphere of cells that forms is known as a **morula**, because it was thought to resemble a mulberry! Each of these new daughter cells is, at this stage, **pluripotential**. In other words, each daughter cell has the potential to differentiate into cells of any lineage.

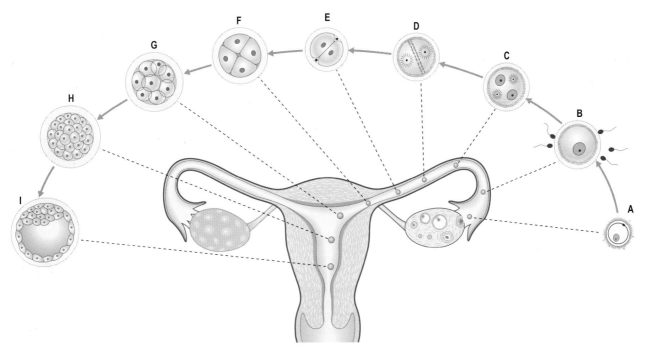

Fig. 1.1 **Stages of pre-embryonic development during the first week.** (**A**) = ovulated oocyte; (**B**) = fertilization; (**C**) = stage of pronuclei formation; (**D**) = first cleavage spindle; (**E–G**) = cleavage of zygote; (**H**) = morula; (**I**) = blastocyst formation.

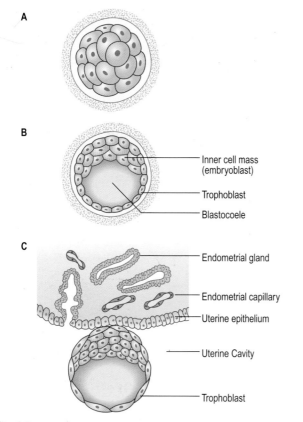

Fig. 1.2 **Early stages of implantation.** A 3-day morula (**A**) and sections of blastocyst are shown at 5 days (**B**) and 6 days (**C**) making contact with the uterine wall.

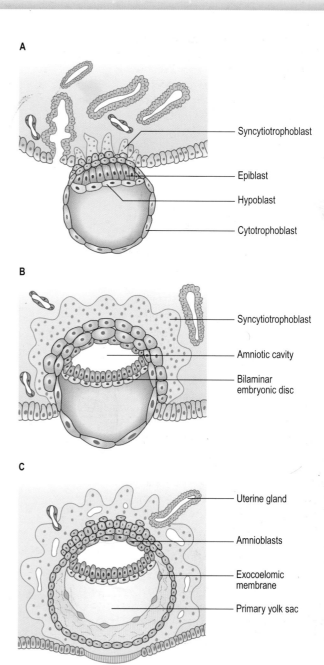

Fig. 1.3 **Implantation of blastocyst.** (**A**) A 7-day blastocyst beginning to implant. (**B**) By 8 days the amniotic cavity appears. (**C**) By 9 days the syncytiotrophoblast invades the uterine glands and capillaries.

. The morula soon shows signs of further differentiation. Cavities appear within the centre of the sphere of cells, forming a **blastocyst**, the cavity itself being the **blastocoele** (Fig. 1.2B,C). Once this stage has been reached the outer layer of the blastocyst soon thins to single-cell thickness to become the **trophoblast**, enclosing the enlarging fluid-filled blastocyst cavity. The central group of cells move to one pole of the blastocyst (the embryonic pole) to form the **inner cell mass** from which the whole embryo itself will form. The trophoblast contributes to the fetal component of the placenta (Fig. 1.3).

The process of morula and blastocyst formation occurs whilst the sphere of dividing cells is in transit along the uterine tube (Fig. 1.1). Fertilization takes place in the **ampulla** of the uterine tube, approximately 12–24 hours after ovulation. The first mitotic division of cleavage will be completed by the time that the two-cell stage embryo

reaches the middle of the tube, at about 30 hours post-fertilization. By 3 days the morula of 12–16 cells will have reached the junction of the uterine tube and the uterus. By 4–5 days the fully formed blastocyst reaches the uterine lumen in preparation for implantation, which occurs a day later.

The 2nd week

Day 8

At this stage the embryo is partly implanted in the endometrium. The implantation process initiates the **decidual reaction** or **decidualization** in the uterine **stroma**, the cells of which contribute the maternal component of the placenta. The trophoblast begins to differentiate: its inner part becomes a single layer of cells,

Clinical box

Abnormal sites of implantation can sometimes occur, due to slow transit of the ovum along the uterine tube. The most common site of **ectopic** implantation is the uterine tube itself, though other sites include the peritoneal cavity or on the surface of the ovary. Such embryos do not come to term because the abnormal implantation site is unable to sustain the developing embryo. Furthermore, the invasive trophoblast tissue causes haemorrhage which can be life-threatening.

hence its name the **cytotrophoblast** (Fig. 1.3A). The outer layer is more extensive and is the invasive layer. It is a **syncytium**, and at this stage, although it has invaded the **endometrium**, it has not invaded endometrial blood vessels. It is known as the **syncytiotrophoblast**. By this stage, the inner cell mass of the blastocyst has differentiated into two layers: the **epiblast** and the **hypoblast** (Fig. 1.3A). These two layers are in contact and form a bilaminar embryonic disc. Within the epiblast a cavity develops, the **amniotic cavity**, which fills with **amniotic fluid**. Some epiblast cells become specialized as **amnioblasts**, and they secrete the amniotic fluid. The **exocoelomic membrane** is derived from the hypoblast and lines the cavity that appears beneath the endoderm, the **primary yolk sac** (Fig. 1.3C). The fluid contained in this sac is the source of nutrition for the embryo before the placenta is fully formed and functional.

By 12 days there has been significant change particularly in the trophoblast. Small clefts appear in the syncytiotrophoblast called **lacunae** which communicate with the maternal endometrial sinusoids, thereby deriving nutritional support for the developing embryo (Fig. 1.4). Concurrent with this is the further development of the cytotrophoblast which is thickest at the embryonic pole of the **conceptus**. Clefts appear between the exocoelomic membrane and the cytotrophoblast (Fig. 1.4). These merge to form the **extra-embryonic coelom** and this cavity comes to almost completely surround the embryo. This is the **chorionic cavity** (Fig. 1.5).

By day 13 the lacunae have enlarged substantially. The cytotrophoblast has begun to form **primary chorionic villi**, which are finger-like protrusions into the lacunae. The embryo proper consists of two layers, the epiblast and the hypoblast, still closely applied to each other. The two cavities continue to enlarge, with the amniotic cavity above the epiblast and the yolk sac below the hypoblast, now known as the **secondary yolk sac** because of the presence of the chorionic cavity (Fig. 1.5). The embryo is connected to the cytotrophoblast by a connecting stalk of extra-embryonic mesoderm (primitive connective tissue) (Fig. 1.5). This stalk

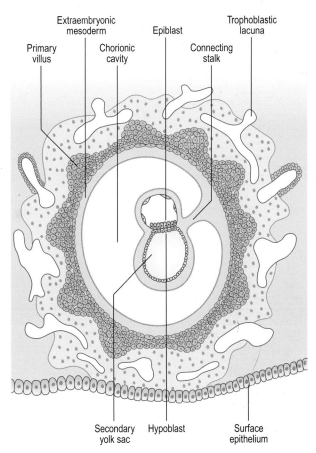

Fig. 1.5 **Formation of chorionic cavity.** At 13 days the germ layers begin to form.

is the forerunner of the umbilical cord. By this stage the uterine epithelium has reformed, thus completely engulfing the conceptus. The largest development of trophoblastic lacunae is on the deepest surface of the conceptus. By the end of the 2nd week the syncytiotrophoblast produces the hormone **human chorionic gonadotrophin** (HCG), which maintains the **corpus luteum** in the ovary, which in turn sustains the thickness of the endometrium. The hormone is secreted in the urine and thus its presence is an early indicator of pregnancy. This is the basis upon which pregnancy test kits work.

Further development of the embryo

The embryo develops further by forming three germ layers, the process known as **gastrulation**. Two layers have already formed: the epiblast and the hypoblast (Fig. 1.5). These two closely apposed layers take up the form of two elliptical plates, and together are termed the **bilaminar embryonic disc**. From this point the epiblast becomes known as the **ectoderm**, and the hypoblast as the **endoderm**. The ectoderm gives rise to the third layer that comes to lie between the two original germ layers, the **intra-embryonic mesoderm**. As a useful generalization, the ectoderm (the outer skin) forms the covering of the body (the epidermis) as well as the nervous system, the endoderm (the inner skin) forms the lining of the gastrointestinal and respiratory systems, and the mesoderm (the middle skin) forms the skeletal, connective and muscle tissues of the body.

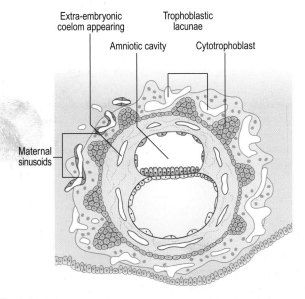

Fig. 1.4 **Implanted blastocyst.** At 12 days cavities develop which coalesce to form the extra-embryonic coelom.

Development of the ectoderm

Primitive streak formation

By the end of the 2nd week of development there is a groove-like midline depression in the **caudal** end of the bilaminar embryonic disc. This marks the appearance of the **primitive streak** (Fig. 1.6). By the beginning of week 3 the streak deepens. At the **cephalic** end of the streak the **primitive node** develops (Fig. 1.6). Cells of the ectoderm layer migrate towards the streak and then detach from it, spreading out laterally beneath it. This migration forms a new germ layer, the intra-embryonic mesoderm. The new germ layer spreads out in all directions to lie between the ectoderm and the endoderm, except in two locations, where the original two germs layers remain in contact: the **prochordal plate**, at the cephalic end of the disc, and the **cloacal plate** at the caudal end of the disc (Fig. 1.7). The prochordal plate is soon replaced by the **buccopharyngeal membrane**, which forms a temporary seal for the future oral cavity. In week 4 this membrane breaks down to establish communication between the gut tube and the amniotic cavity. The cloacal plate is replaced by the cloacal membrane.

Notochord formation

Cells derived from the primitive node migrate cranially towards the buccopharyngeal membrane (Fig. 1.7). This results in the appearance of the **notochordal plate**, which in turn folds in to form the solid cylinder of the **notochord**. The notochord thus comes to underlie the future neural tube (the future brain and spinal cord–see below and Chapter 10), and forms both a longitudinal axis for the embryo, and the centres (nuclei pulposi) of the intervertebral discs of the vertebral column.

Neurulation

The process of the formation of the brain and spinal cord is known as **neurulation**. The ectoderm germ layer gives rise

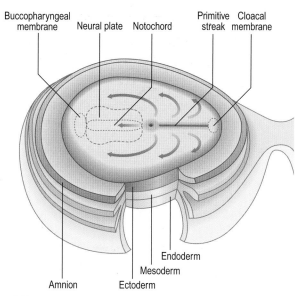

Fig. 1.7 **Dorsal view of the embryonic disc showing the formation of the notochord.** By day 18 the notochord induces the overlying ectoderm to form the neural plate. Arrows indicate the migration of intra-embryonic mesoderm.

to **neuroectoderm**, which gives rise to most of the major components of the nervous system. At about 19 days, at the cranial end of the primitive streak, the underlying mesoderm and notochord induce the ectoderm to form the **neural plate** (Fig. 1.7), which rounds up to form the neural folds (Fig. 1.8A,B). The neural plate enlarges initially at the cranial end. At 20 days, the neural plate in the mid-region of the embryo remains narrowed, but it expands at the caudal end. The plate deepens to form the **neural groove** from which the **neural tube** forms. The cranial and caudal ends of the tube are open and are known as the **anterior** and **posterior neuropores**; these eventually close (Fig. 1.8C,D). At the edges of the neural tube, where the neuroectoderm is continuous with the surface ectoderm, the **neural crests** are formed. The neural crest cells detach themselves from the rest of the neural groove, before the tube forms, forming discrete aggregations of neural crest cells (Fig. 1.9). They contribute to the formation of dorsal root, cranial, enteric and autonomic ganglia, connective tissues of the face and bones of the skull, the adrenal medulla, glial cells, Schwann cells, melanocytes, parts of the meninges and parts of teeth. The further development of the nervous system will be dealt with in Chapter 10.

Further development of the mesoderm

As the numbers of cells increase each side of the notochord, by day 17 the layer is thickest closest to the midline, and is known as the **paraxial mesoderm**. The parts further out are known as the **intermediate** and **lateral plate mesoderm** (Fig. 1.9C). At day 19, clefts begin to appear in the lateral plate. The mesoderm of the lateral plate is continuous with the extra-embryonic mesoderm covering the amniotic sac and the yolk sac (Fig. 1.9A,B). The mesoderm covering the amniotic sac is termed the parietal or somatic layer and that covering the yolk sac the visceral or splanchnic layer (Fig. 1.9B). The diverging limbs of the extra-embryonic mesoderm open into the extra-embryonic coelom (space or cavity). The clefts that appear within the lateral plate merge to form the **intra-embryonic coelom**, a

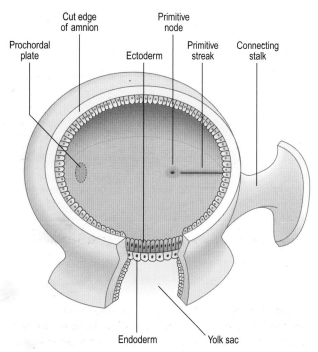

Fig. 1.6 **Dorsal view of a 15-day embryonic disc after removal of part of the amniotic sac revealing the primitive node and primitive streak.**

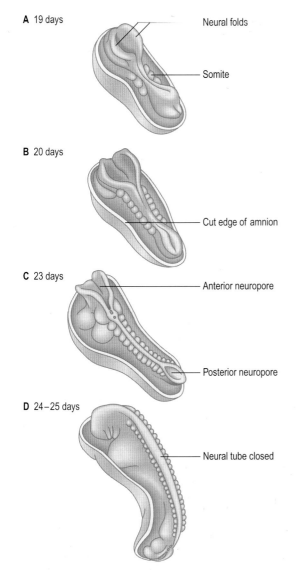

A 19 days — Neural folds
— Somite

B 20 days — Cut edge of amnion

C 23 days — Anterior neuropore
— Posterior neuropore

D 24–25 days — Neural tube closed

Fig. 1.8 **Formation of the neural tube between days 19 and 25 after removal of part of the amniotic sac.** The neural folds first fuse in the head and cervical region. The anterior and posterior neuropores close between days 24 and 25.

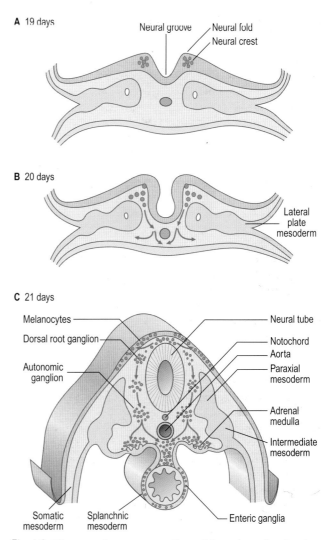

A 19 days — Neural groove — Neural fold — Neural crest

B 20 days — Lateral plate mesoderm

C 21 days
Melanocytes — Neural tube
Dorsal root ganglion — Notochord
— Aorta
Autonomic ganglion — Paraxial mesoderm
— Adrenal medulla
— Intermediate mesoderm
Somatic mesoderm — Splanchnic mesoderm — Enteric ganglia

Fig. 1.9 **Diagrams of transverse sections of the embryo showing the origin and migration of neural crest cells between days 19 and 21.**

cavity which is the forerunner of the serous cavities (Fig. 1.10) (i.e. the pericardial, pleural and peritoneal cavities). The intra-embryonic and extra-embryonic coeloms are therefore continuous.

Arising between the paraxial and lateral plate mesoderm is the intermediate mesoderm from which the urogenital system develops (Fig. 1.9C) (see Chapters 8 and 9).

Segmentation of the mesoderm

Paraxial mesoderm
The paraxial mesoderm undergoes further differentiation in paired blocks of tissue in a craniocaudal direction on each side of the notochord called **somites.** The first pair of somites form at about 20 days, and thereafter at a rate of about three per day until 42–44 pairs are formed, though not all persist into adulthood. The age of an embryo is related to the number of somite pairs present. From the beginning of the 4th week the somites undergo further differentiation to form **dermomyotomes** (form connective tissue and skeletal muscle) and **sclerotomes** (form bone

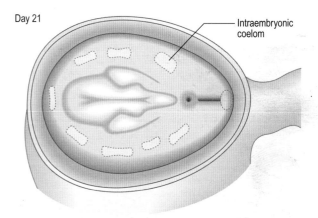

Day 21 — Intraembryonic coelom

Fig. 1.10 **Diagram of a 21-day embryo showing the formation of intra-embryonic coelom after removal of part of the amniotic sac.**

and cartilage) (Fig. 1.11A). Cells from the sclerotomes surround the notochord and spinal cord, and give rise to the vertebral column. Details of the formation of vertebrae, and the contribution made by the sclerotomes, may be found in Chapter 4.

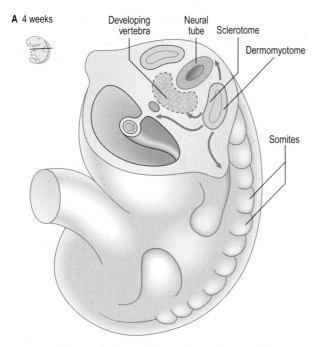

A 4 weeks
Developing vertebra
Neural tube
Sclerotome
Dermomyotome
Somites

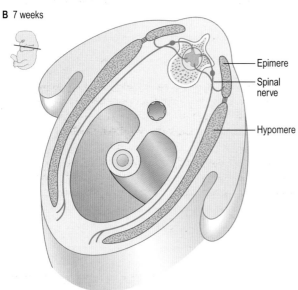

B 7 weeks
Epimere
Spinal nerve
Hypomere

Fig. 1.11 (**A**) Subdivisions of the somite by 4 weeks. Arrows indicate the migration of somitic mesodermal cells. (**B**) The origin of segmental musculature from dermomyotome at 7 weeks by splitting of myotome into a dorsal epimere and ventral hypomere.

Somite development

In the 4th week, the medially placed mesenchymal cells of the somites migrate towards the notochord to form sclerotomes (**mesenchyme** is the loosely arranged embryonic connective tissue in the embryo). The ventrolateral cells of the somites become the myotomes, and those remaining become the dermatomes (Fig. 1.11A). The myotomes split into dorsal **epimeres** and ventral **hypomeres**. The dorsal epimeres give rise to **epaxial** muscles, the erector spinae muscles. The ventral hypomeres give rise to **hypaxial** muscles which include muscles of the body wall (Fig. 1.11B). The ventrolateral parts of the somites in the regions of the future limb buds that remain after the sclerotomal portion has formed migrate to differentiate into limb musculature (see Chapter 4). The dermatomes form the dermis of the skin, and thus these cells come to lie

beneath the surface ectoderm, which forms the uppermost layer of the skin, the epidermis. It is important to appreciate that as the myotomes and dermatomes migrate to their adult position they bring with them their innervation, from the segment of origin of the developing spinal cord.

The lateral plate mesoderm

The two layers of the lateral plate mesoderm enclose the intra-embryonic coelom. The mesodermal cells of the lateral plate arrange themselves as thin layers, which become the serous membranes of the body: the **pleura**, **pericardium** and **peritoneum.** These two continuous layers differentiate therefore to become a lining for the future body wall, a covering for the future endodermal gut tube (see Chapter 7) and the smooth muscle and connective tissue of the gut wall. The development of the body cavities is dealt with in Chapter 3. The serous layer in contact with the future body

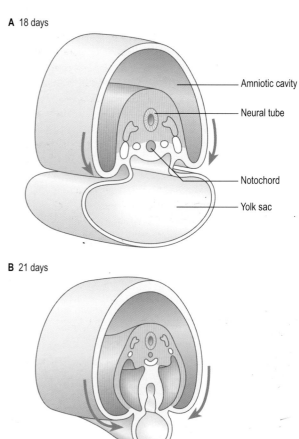

A 18 days
Amniotic cavity
Neural tube
Notochord
Yolk sac

B 21 days

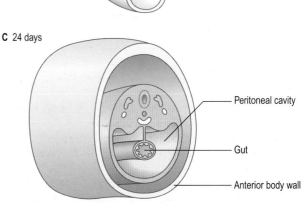

C 24 days
Peritoneal cavity
Gut
Anterior body wall

Fig. 1.12 **Formation of the lateral body folds between 18 and 21 days in transverse sections of the embryo.** Arrows indicate the lateral folds. By 24 days lateral folding is complete.

wall is the **parietal** layer because **parietes** means wall in Latin; the serous layer in contact with the endodermal gut tube, for instance, is the **visceral** layer because **viscera** means organs. Other names for these two layers are **somatopleure** (meaning membrane associated with the body side) and **splanchnopleure** (meaning membrane associated with the organ side) (Fig. 1.9B).

The endoderm

The epithelial lining of the gastrointestinal tract is derived from the endoderm germ layer. The formation of the endodermal gut tube depends on the **transverse** and **longitudinal folding** of the embryo. In addition to the lining of the gastrointestinal and respiratory systems, the endoderm also gives rise to the **parenchymal** cells of the liver and pancreas (see Chapter 7), and of the thyroid and parathyroids, as well as the lining of the urinary bladder.

Folding of the embryo

Folding takes place in two directions: **longitudinal** (also referred to as **cephalocaudal**) and **lateral** (or **transverse**). Longitudinal folding occurs mainly as a consequence of the rapid enlargement of the cranial end of the neural tube to form the brain (see Chapter 10). Lateral folding is a consequence of the enlargement of the somites. The process of lateral folding is illustrated in Figure 1.12.

Longitudinal folding, which occurs between days 21 and 24, results in bending of the embryo so that the head and tail are brought closer together (Fig. 1.13). The endoderm forms a tube-like structure with an initially wide communication with the yolk sac: this communication narrows as the longitudinal folding increases. The amniotic cavity pushes in at the cranial and caudal ends of the

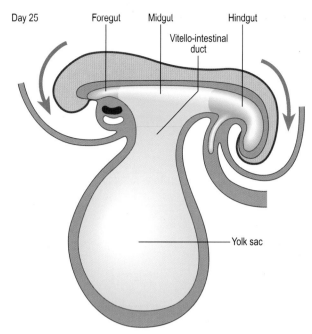

Fig. 1.13 **The process of longitudinal folding by day 25 in a sagittal section of an embryo.** Arrows indicate the formation of head and tail folds.

embryonic disc, thus increasing the degree of longitudinal folding at the head and tail folds. The amniotic cavity also pinches the connection of the yolk sac and gut to form the narrowed communication of the **vitello-intestinal** (or **vitelline**) duct (Fig. 1.13). Later this duct is lost.

In humans the yolk sac plays a role in the early nutrition of the embryo, but this is lost after the first month or so, and a vestigial yolk sac lies freely in the chorionic cavity.

Summary box

- The series of rapid mitotic divisions of the ovum result in the formation of a morula, and then a blastocyst. The blastocyst is a fluid-filled hollow sphere, which consists of an inner cell mass at one pole, surrounded by a thin wall of trophoblast cells.
- The trophoblast cells attach the blastocyst to the uterine wall, and form the fetal portion of the placenta.
- The trophoblast differentiates into syncytiotrophoblast and cytotrophoblast. Lacunae appear in the syncytiotrophoblast, and merge to communicate with maternal blood sinusoids. By this the embryo derives nutrition from the maternal circulation. The cytotrophoblast forms villi, which are finger-like protrusions into the lacunae.
- The amniotic and chorionic cavities come to surround the embryo and their walls constitute the fetal membranes.
- The endometrium responds to implantation by mounting the decidual reaction. The decidua basalis forms the maternal component of the placenta.
- The inner cell mass differentiates into two of the three primary germ layers: the epiblast (later the ectoderm) and the hypoblast (later the endoderm). This process is known as gastrulation, and results in a bilaminar embryonic disc.

- The ectoderm further differentiates and forms the primitive streak which gives rise to the third germ layer, the mesoderm. Thus, the trilaminar embryonic disc forms. The mesoderm differentiates further into paraxial, intermediate and lateral plate mesoderm. The lateral plate mesoderm encloses the intra-embryonic coelom.
- The paraxial mesoderm forms the segmented somites, which give rise to muscles, skeletal structures and dermis. The intermediate mesoderm contributes to the urogenital system, and the lateral plate mesoderm forms the parietal and visceral layers of the serous membranes of the body.
- Neurulation is the process by which the ectoderm gives rise to the neural tube and neural crests of the developing brain and spinal cord.
- At the cranial end of the primitive streak, at the primitive node, the notochord forms, and this grows cranially and constitutes a midline axis of the body: it largely disappears before birth, but persists as the centres of the intervertebral discs of the vertebral column.
- The endoderm gives rise to the linings of the gastrointestinal and respiratory systems, and of the urinary bladder, as well as the parenchyma of the liver and pancreas.
- The trilaminar disc undergoes longitudinal and lateral folding, thus forming the folded embryo.

Chapter 2
How do the placenta and fetal membranes form?

During fertilization and initial formation of the blastocyst the early embryo receives its nutrition by diffusion through the **zona pellucida** from the accumulated fluid found in the blastocoele. However, after the blastocyst has hatched from the zona pellucida, allowing attachment to the uterine epithelium on the 5th or 6th day after fertilization, the embryo grows faster, thus the need for a more efficient method of nutrition becomes essential. From 12 days until full term, the developing embryo and fetus obtain their nutrition from maternal blood. This is achieved by the formation of a placenta and the development of the **uteroplacental circulation**.

In response to the circulating progesterone and to the blastocyst, the stromal cells of the endometrium become large and accumulate glycogen. At 12 days the syncytiotrophoblast of the blastocyst begins to erode the endometrium and the maternal vessels at the implantation site become congested and dilated. These cellular changes, together with an increase in endometrial vascularization, are known as the **decidual reaction**. Within a few days the decidual reaction spreads throughout the endometrium, which now is known as the decidua. As the implanted embryo bulges into the uterine lumen the decidua becomes identifiable as three discrete areas at the implantation site (Fig. 2.1). The decidua underlying the embryo is called the **decidua basalis**, which forms the maternal face of the placenta. The **decidua capsularis** lines the superficial part of the embryo bulging into the uterine lumen and the remainder of the decidua is called the **decidua parietalis**.

What are the fetal membranes?

The term fetal membrane is applied to those structures derived from the blastocyst which do not contribute to the embryo. The **amnion**, the **chorion**, the **yolk sac** and the **allantois** make up the fetal membranes (Fig. 2.2). The amnion lines the amniotic sac and protects the embryo from physical injury. The chorion is a double-layered membrane

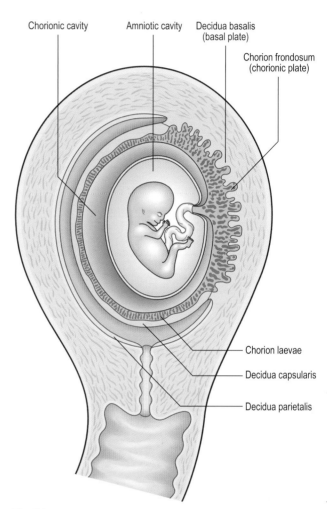

Fig. 2.1 **Development of the deciduae at 12 weeks.**

formed by the trophoblast and the extra-embryonic mesoderm, which eventually will give rise to the fetal part of the placenta. From 12 days until the end of embryonic period the developing embryo is suspended in the chorionic cavity. The only connection between the embryo and the chorion is via a thick plate of mesoderm called the connecting stalk.

The yolk sac and its diverticulum, the allantois, are the major means of nutritional exchange mechanisms in other mammals. However, in humans the yolk reserves are poor, and part of the yolk sac is incorporated into the embryo to form the gut tube. The allantois, which serves as a reservoir for fetal urine in other mammals, becomes attached to the urinary bladder.

A 10-day implantation site

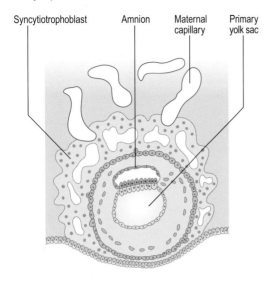

Syncytiotrophoblast · Amnion · Maternal capillary · Primary yolk sac

B 15-day implantation site

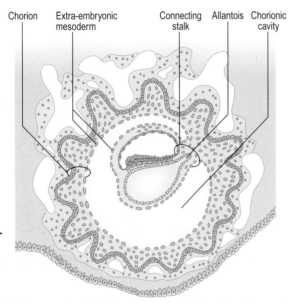

Chorion · Extra-embryonic mesoderm · Connecting stalk · Allantois · Chorionic cavity

Fig. 2.2 **Formation of fetal membranes at implantation sites at 10 days (A) and 15 days (B).**

A

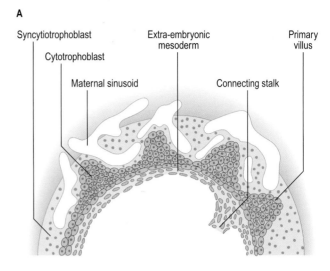

Syncytiotrophoblast · Cytotrophoblast · Maternal sinusoid · Extra-embryonic mesoderm · Connecting stalk · Primary villus

B

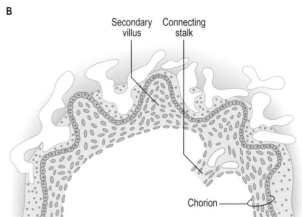

Secondary villus · Connecting stalk · Chorion

Fig. 2.3 **Function of the chorionic villi. (A)** By day 14, the primary villi appear as cytotrophoblastic stems. **(B)** By day 16, the extra-embryonic mesoderm grows into the villi, thus transforming each primary villus into a secondary villus.

Development of the uteroplacental circulation

Due to the rapid growth of the embryo during the 2nd week, there is a need for a more efficient means of nutritional and gaseous exchange. This is achieved when the embryonic blood vessels of the chorion come into contact with the maternal blood vessels of the decidua.

The **umbilical arteries** carry the deoxygenated blood from the embryo to the chorion and **umbilical veins** return the oxygenated blood to the embryo. The uterine vessels supply the maternal blood to the trophoblastic lacunae. When the cytotrophoblast cells grow into the lacunae as the primary chorionic villi, the primitive uteroplacental circulation is established. The initial formation of primary chorionic villi is explained in Chapter 1.

Further development of chorionic villi

From day 15, the **primary chorionic villi** begin to branch, and the extra-embryonic (chorionic) mesoderm invades the core of the primary villi, thus converting them into **secondary chorionic villi** (Fig. 2.3). The secondary villi line the entire surface of the chorion, and soon blood vessels develop within the mesenchyme of these villi that connect to the umbilical vessels in the embryo. Villi containing blood vessels are called **tertiary villi** (Fig. 2.4).

As the embryo and its coverings grow, the chorionic villi on the **abembryonic pole** become compressed against the decidua capsularis and become avascular (Figs 2.1, 2.5). This area of chorion is known as the smooth chorion or **chorion laeve**. As the chorion laeve regresses, the villi on the embryonic pole increase in size and number. Because of its leafy appearance, this portion of the chorion is known as the **chorion frondosum** (Figs 2.1, 2.5).

Formation of the placenta and placental circulation

The placenta has both maternal and fetal components. The maternal portion is called the **basal plate** and is derived from

A

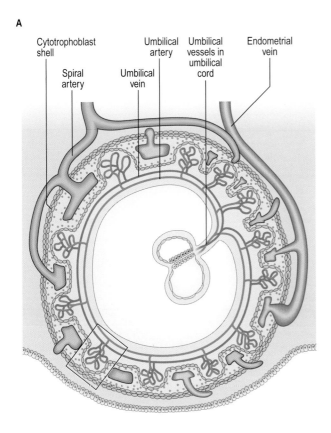

B

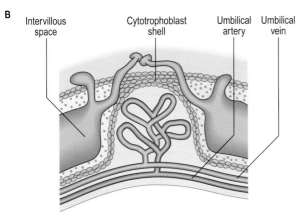

Fig. 2.4 **By day 21, blood vessels develop within the chorionic mesoderm forming the tertiary villi.** (**B**) Enlarged view of boxed area in (**A**) showing a tertiary villus.

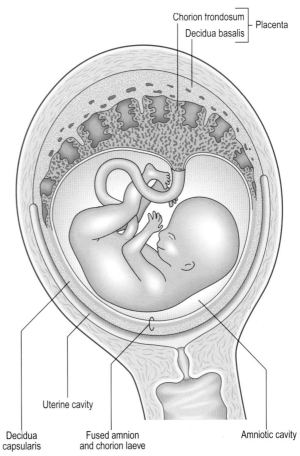

Fig. 2.5 **Fetus at the end of the 3rd month showing the fused amnion and chorion laeve.** The placenta is formed by the decidua basalis and chorion frondosum.

the decidua basalis, and the fetal portion is called the **chorionic plate**, formed by the chorion frondosum (Fig. 2.1). The tertiary villi of the chorion frondosum grow towards the basal plate, and attach to the decidual tissue via the **cytotrophoblast shell** (Fig. 2.4B). Because these villi secure the attachment of the fetal placenta to the basal plate, they are known as **anchoring villi** (Fig. 2.6A). The blood-filled spaces between the anchoring villi, which were trophoblastic lacunae, now become the **intervillous spaces** (Fig. 2.6A).

The anchoring villi give rise to numerous side branches called **intermediate villi**, which in turn produce small rounded **terminal** or **floating villi** (Fig. 2.7). The terminal villi develop as sprouts of syncytiotrophoblast. During the third trimester, the terminal villi take over the functions of nutrient and gaseous exchange from the intermediate villi. The continuous branching of the villi into the intervillous spaces therefore results in an extensive placental villous tree.

As the placenta grows during the last trimester of pregnancy, the placental villi show maturation changes. The capillaries become larger and come to lie close to a much thinner syncytiotrophoblast. Most of the cells of the cytotrophoblast layer disappear, thus facilitating diffusional exchange mechanisms.

As the villous trees grow into the intervillous spaces, the decidual tissue sends wedge-like **placental septa** to divide the placenta into 15–20 irregular convex areas called **cotyledons**. Since the placental septa do not reach the chorionic plate, the maternal circulation between the cotyledons is maintained (Fig. 2.6A).

The exchange of nutrients, respiratory gases and waste products between the maternal and fetal blood takes place across the **placental membrane** (see below) within the intervillous spaces. Maternal blood enters these spaces from the **spiral arteries**, branches of the uterine artery, bringing nutrients and oxygen for the embryo and fetus, and the **endometrial veins** drain the waste products to the maternal circulation (Figs 2.4A, 2.6A). The oxygenated fetal blood from the placenta passes into the umbilical vein, and the deoxygenated blood from the fetus is returned to the placenta by way of the umbilical arteries.

Placental membrane and placental functions

The partition between the maternal and fetal circulations is the placental membrane, often called the placental barrier

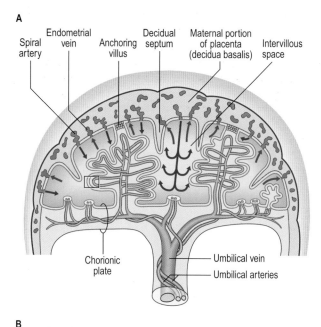

A

- Spiral artery
- Endometrial vein
- Anchoring villus
- Decidual septum
- Maternal portion of placenta (decidua basalis)
- Intervillous space
- Chorionic plate
- Umbilical vein
- Umbilical arteries

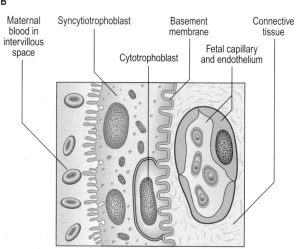

B

- Maternal blood in intervillous space
- Syncytiotrophoblast
- Cytotrophoblast
- Basement membrane
- Fetal capillary and endothelium
- Connective tissue

Fig. 2.6 **The full-term placenta showing the maternal and fetal portions (A).** The decidual septa divide the maternal portion into cotyledons. Arrows indicate the direction of maternal blood flow. The boxed area is enlarged in (**B**). Placental membrane (**B**).

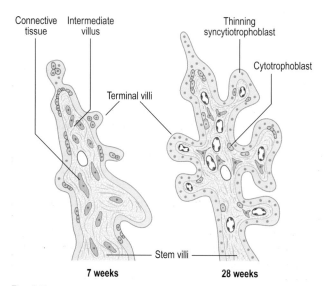

- Connective tissue
- Intermediate villus
- Terminal villi
- Thinning syncytiotrophoblast
- Cytotrophoblast
- Stem villi

7 weeks   28 weeks

Fig. 2.7 **Maturation of placental villi at 7 and 28 weeks.**

(Fig. 2.6B). This membrane is composed of fetal tissues and is initially four layers thick: (1) the fetal capillary endothelium, (2) the connective tissue of the villus, (3) the cytotrophoblast and (4) the syncytiotrophoblast. From the 4th month the placental membrane becomes progressively thinner as the fetal capillaries enlarge, the amount of connective tissue in the core of the villus is reduced, and the cytotrophoblast largely disappears.

The most important function of the placenta is to provide exchange of nutrients and waste products between the mother and fetus. The surface of the syncytiotrophoblast facing the intervillous spaces shows numerous microvilli, and these increase the area available for physiological exchange. Smaller molecules are transmitted by simple diffusion, but for larger molecules mechanisms of either active transport or pinocytosis are involved. Maternal antibodies cross the placental membrane by pinocytosis, and these give passive immunity to the newborn. Another important function of the placenta is that of secretion of hormones. The trophoblast secretes HCG, which maintains the corpus luteum. The placenta also produces large amounts of progesterone and oestrogen.

Structure of the full-term placenta

At term the placenta appears as a disc, and has fetal and maternal surfaces (Fig. 2.8). The **fetal surface** is smooth, and the **umbilical cord** is inserted into the centre of this surface. The amnion invests the umbilical cord, and covers the fetal surface of the placenta. The umbilical vessels radiate from the umbilical cord, and run between the transparent amnion and smooth chorion before supplying the chorionic villi. At birth the amnion and chorion are torn from the margins of the placenta. The **maternal surface** is covered by a thin layer of decidua basalis torn from the uterine wall during birth. Beneath this layer, the maternal surface shows 15–20 roughened cotyledons (Fig. 2.8A).

> ### Clinical box
> **Erythroblastosis fetalis**
> Passage of fetal red blood cells across the placenta normally occurs without problem, but this transfer may sometimes be fatal. If the fetal red blood cells containing Rhesus (Rh) positive surface molecules cross the placental membrane into the Rh negative mother, the anti-Rh antibodies produced by the mother pass to the fetal blood vessels which results in destruction of the fetal red blood cells. Fetuses with this condition, called haemolytic disease of the newborn or erythroblastosis fetalis, may die in severe cases unless given intra-uterine Rh negative blood transfusions.
>
> **Transmission of viral and bacterial infections**
> The survival of the fetus is at risk when the mother is infected with viral or bacterial organisms. In the first 3 months of pregnancy rubella viruses may pass through the placenta and cause congenital abnormalities of the eye and the heart. The bacterium which causes maternal syphilis may cross the placental membrane. Human immunodeficiency virus (HIV) present in the maternal blood can sometimes cross the placenta to infect the fetus.

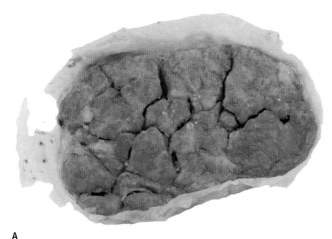

A

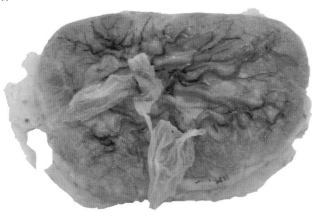

B

Fig. 2.8 **Photograph of a full-term placenta. (A)** Maternal surface. **(B)** Fetal surface.

Following the delivery of the child at birth, the placenta separates from the uterine wall and is expelled by uterine contractions through the cervix.

The umbilical cord

The umbilical cord suspends the embryo in the amniotic cavity. The cord contains two umbilical arteries and one umbilical vein through which blood passes between the embryo and the placenta. The umbilical vessels are surrounded by mucoid tissue, called Wharton's jelly. Within the umbilical cord the arteries coil around the single vein giving the umbilical cord a spiral twist appearance.

Clinical box
Attachment of placenta
The commonest site of placental attachment is on the upper posterior wall of the uterus. However, it may attach at any place on the uterine wall. If the blastocyst implants at a lower level in the uterus, **placenta previa** develops near the internal os of the cervix. This may result in uterine bleeding before birth and premature separation of the placenta, and in 15–20% of such cases the infant may not survive.

Clinical box
Knots in the umbilical cord
The umbilical cord may show **true** or **false knots**. The false knots occur because the umbilical vessels are longer than the cord, and these are of no significance. True knots may occur when the fetus passes through the loop of the cord, but they rarely tighten to interfere with the fetal circulation.

Twins and their fetal membranes

The organization of fetal membranes in twins depends on the type of twins and on the stage of development at which the original single embryo separates. Two types of twins occur: **dizygotic** and **monozygotic**. Dizygotic or non-identical twins result when the two released oocytes fertilize with two different spermatozoa. Twins that form by the splitting of a single zygote are called monozygotic or identical twins.

Dizygotic twins implant separately and develop separate placentae and fetal membranes (Fig. 2.9A). Sometimes, however, because of their proximity a secondary fusion between the two amniotic and chorionic sacs may occur.

The sharing of placenta and fetal membranes in monozygotic twins depends on the stage at which a single zygote divides. If the splitting occurs at the two-cell stage of the embryo, the resulting twins will implant separately with their own fetal membranes and placentae (Fig. 9B). In such cases, although the arrangement of fetal membranes is the same as that of the non-identical dizygotic twins, their identity as monozygotic twins can only be revealed by conducting blood and other diagnostic tests. In most cases of identical twinning, the inner cell mass splits within a single blastocyst. Subsequently, two embryos will share a single chorionic sac and placenta but will be enclosed by separate amniotic sacs (Fig. 9B). If the splitting occurs after the formation of the bilaminar embryonic disc, the twins will occupy a single amnion and chorionic sac, and share the same placenta (Fig. 9C). Such twins usually fail to survive, as the umbilical cords may get entangled within the amniotic sac thus blocking the fetal circulation.

Summary box

- The placenta develops from both maternal and fetal tissues to provide nutrients and oxygen to the fetus, and carry waste products to the mother.
- The maternal and fetal circulations are separated by a placental membrane derived from fetal tissues.
- The umbilical cord connects the placenta to the embryo.
- The chorion and amnion become fused around the fully formed placenta.
- The extent to which the fetal membranes are shared in twins depends on their derivation and the time at which the separation of embryonic cells occurs.

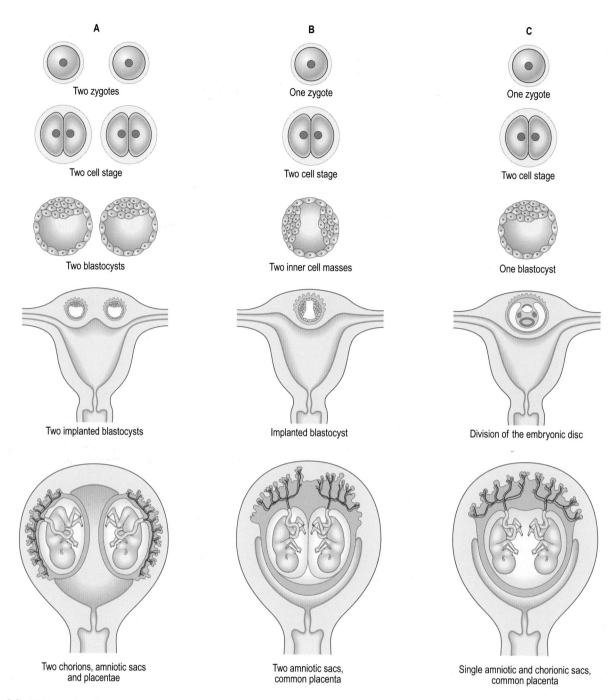

A

Two zygotes

Two cell stage

Two blastocysts

Two implanted blastocysts

Two chorions, amniotic sacs
and placentae

B

One zygote

Two cell stage

Two inner cell masses

Implanted blastocyst

Two amniotic sacs,
common placenta

C

One zygote

Two cell stage

One blastocyst

Division of the embryonic disc

Single amniotic and chorionic sacs,
common placenta

Fig. 2.9 **(A) Dizygotic twins.** (**B**) Monozygotic twinning resulting from the splitting of inner cell mass (**C**) Monozygotic twinning resulting from the splitting of embryonic disc.

Chapter 3
The body cavities and the diaphragm

The embryo takes on a three-dimensional shape during the 4th week when the edges of the embryonic disc are brought to the ventral surface of the embryo by lateral and longitudinal folding. Folding of the embryo results in the formation of the gut tube and converts the **intra-embryonic coelom** into a closed cavity. The process of folding is described in Chapter 1.

The **body cavities** arise from the three parts of the coelomic cavity, and become the future pericardial, pleural and peritoneal cavities. Delicate **serous membranes**, derived from the lateral plate mesoderm, line the walls of those cavities and cover the organs. The main function of the body cavities is to provide space for development, expansion and movement of organs such as heart, lungs and liver. The body cavities are lined by two serous layers: the **somatic mesoderm**, which is in contact with the **ectoderm**, and the **splanchnic mesoderm** which adheres to the endoderm (see Fig 1.9C). The term somatic refers to the body wall; therefore the somatic mesoderm will give rise to the parietal layer of the serous membranes. The term splanchnic is used for organs, and the splanchnic mesoderm will form the visceral layer of serous membranes.

Septum transversum and intra-embryonic coelom

Before folding
The **septum transversum** is a sheet of mesoderm that appears on day 22 **rostral** to the developing heart (Fig. 3.1).

Clinical box
Gastroschisis
When an infant is born with a defect in the anterior abdominal wall this may allow the abdominal contents to protrude outside the body. Unlike an omphalocoele (see Chapter 7), the protruding intestines are not covered by peritoneum or amnion. Gastroschisis may happen when the lateral folds of the embryo fail to meet in the midline. The abnormality may also occur due to deficiency of somatic mesoderm and its incomplete migration to the anterior abdominal wall.

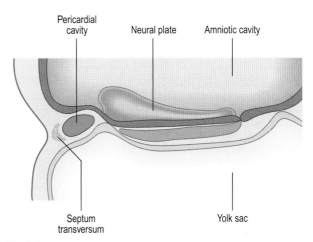
Fig. 3.1 **Sagittal section of a 3-week embryo showing the position of the septum transversum rostral to the pericardial cavity.**

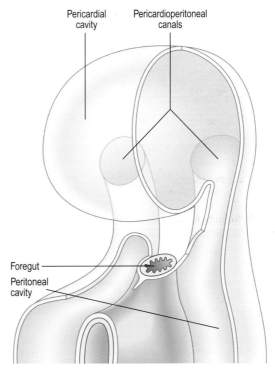
Fig. 3.2 **The ventrolateral view of the intra-embryonic coelom in a 4-week embryo.**

Before folding, the intra-embryonic coelom appears as a horseshoe- or U-shaped cavity (Fig. 3.2). The bend of the U lies anteriorly, and represents the part of the coelomic cavity from which the **pericardial cavity** will develop. Each limb of the U consists of two cavities: (1) a **pericardioperitoneal**

canal, from which the pleural cavity will develop, and (2) a **peritoneal cavity** which lies in the future abdomen. In the umbilical region, the peritoneal cavities in each limb open into the chorionic cavity or the extra-embryonic coelom. This communication allows the herniation of midgut loops into the umbilical cord (see Chapter 7).

After folding

As a result of the head fold, the heart, with its pericardial cavity, swings ventral to the foregut. The septum transversum, initially cranial to the pericardial cavity, finally is wedged between the heart and the neck of the yolk sac. The pericardial cavity now opens into the paired pericardioperitoneal canals, which run on either side of the foregut to reach the peritoneal cavity. These canals end in two openings on the dorsolateral aspect of the foregut, therefore, at this stage the septum transversum is an incomplete partition between the thorax and abdomen (Fig. 3.3). The septum transversum forms the central tendon of the diaphragm.

Division of the intra-embryonic coelom into four cavities

Paired **mesenchymal** ridges grow from the lateral body wall into the pericardioperitoneal canals and separate these paired cavities from the pericardial and peritoneal cavities (Fig. 3.4). When invaginated by the lung buds, the pericardioperitoneal canals become the pleural cavities. The **pleuropericardial folds** separate the pleural cavity from the pericardial cavity, and the more substantial caudal partitions, which separate the pleural cavity from the peritoneal cavity, are known as the **pleuroperitoneal membranes**. The pleuroperitoneal membranes are at the level of the septum transversum.

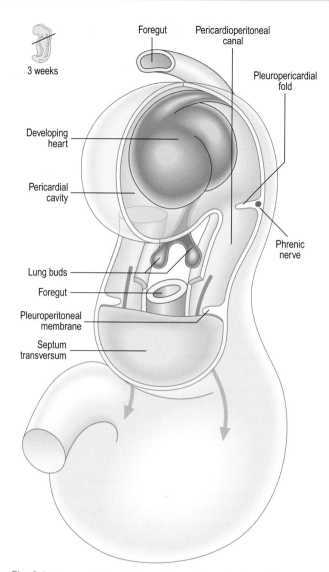

Fig. 3.4 **The ventrolateral view of the embryo showing the pericardial cavity, pericardioperitoneal canals and their associated folds and membranes.** The arrows indicate communication between the pericardioperitoneal canals and the peritoneal cavity.

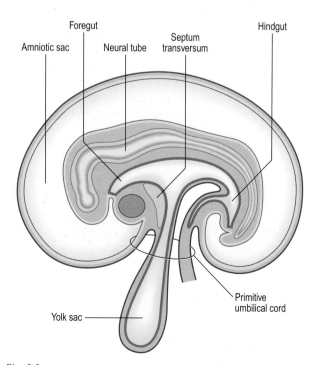

Fig. 3.3 **Longitudinal section of a 25-day embryo showing the head and tail folds.** Note the position of the septum transversum between the pericardial cavity and the yolk sac.

As the heart descends, the pleuropericardial folds migrate ventrally and fuse with each other forming the **fibrous pericardium**. The thoracic cavity is then divided into a definitive pericardial cavity and two lateral pleural cavities. The **phrenic nerves**, which have been located within the pleuropericardial folds, run through the fibrous pericardium in the adult to supply the diaphragm.

The diaphragm

Initially, the septum transversum forms an incomplete partition between the thoracic and abdominal cavities, due to the presence of the pericardioperitoneal canals. Soon a number of mesodermal structures fuse with each other at the level of the septum transversum to form the definitive diaphragm. Five structures, described below, contribute to the development of the diaphragm (Fig. 3.5).

The septum transversum

The septum transversum, composed of mesoderm, gives rise to the central tendon of the diaphragm.

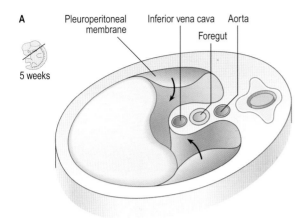

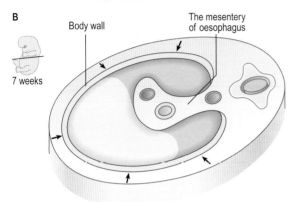

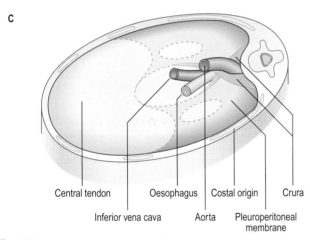

Fig. 3.5 **Formation of the diaphragm as seen from above. (A)** At week 5 the pleuroperitoneal membranes are growing towards the septum transversum. (**B**) At week 7 the membranes have fused with the septum transversum. Note the arrows indicating ingrowth of the body wall (**C**) the components of the diaphragm in a newborn. The outlines of the pleuroperitoneal canals may still be seen, and are the potential sites of congenital defects.

The body wall

As the pleural cavities enlarge and extend into the lateral body walls, the somatic mesoderm contributes to the outer rim of the diaphragm. Extensions of the pleural cavities form the costodiaphragmatic recesses. The peripheral part of the diaphragm attached to the ribs, therefore, receives its sensory innervation from the lower six intercostal nerves.

The mesentery of the oesophagus

The mesenchyme around the oesophagus and its mesentery contribute to the connective tissues of the diaphragm. During further development, the muscular crura of the diaphragm are formed as mesenchymal condensations within the mesentery of the oesophagus.

The pleuroperitoneal membranes

These membranes fuse with the mesentery of the oesophagus and with the septum transversum, thus sealing off the pleural cavities from the peritoneal cavity. The pleuroperitoneal membranes contribute a small portion to the fully developed diaphragm.

The cervical somites

During the 4th week, the heart and septum transversum lie in the cervical region opposite the 3rd, 4th and 5th cervical somites. At this stage the myoblasts from these somites migrate into the septum transversum and differentiate into the diaphragmatic musculature. Because of its origin the muscle of the diaphragm is innervated by the nerves of 3rd, 4th and 5th segments of the cervical spinal cord. The nerve fibres from these segments join to form the phrenic nerve. The final thoracic position of the diaphragm is reached during the 6th week after descent of the heart and formation of the neck. This accounts for the cervical origin of the nerves supplying the diaphragm.

> ### Clinical box
> **Diaphragmatic herniae**
> If one of the pleuroperitoneal canals fails to close, the abdominal viscera may enter the pleural cavity (Fig. 3.6). This condition, called a diaphragmatic hernia, is usually on the left side. Because of the presence of the abdominal viscera in the chest, the heart is displaced, and the lungs are reduced in size. Consequently, the affected child may have severe respiratory problems even after the hernia is surgically repaired.
>
> Sometimes, congenital herniae occur through small gaps in the anterior part of the diaphragm near its sternal attachment or through the oesophageal opening. These herniae, known as the **parasternal** and **oesophageal hernia** respectively, do not usually have any clinical significance. Acquired diaphragmatic herniae usually occur through the oesophageal opening and are termed **hiatal herniae**. Such herniae may have a peritoneal covering, and be associated with digestive disturbances.

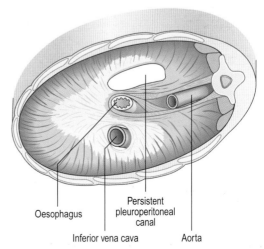

Fig. 3.6 **A left postero-lateral defect in the diaphragm seen in a newborn from below.**

Summary box

- The space formed within the lateral plate mesoderm becomes the intra-embryonic coelom lined by the somatic and visceral layers of lateral plate mesoderm.
- The somatic mesodermal layer becomes the parietal serous membrane and the splanchnic mesodermal layer becomes the visceral serous membrane.
- After folding of the embryo, partitions divide this coelom into pericardial, pleural and peritoneal cavities.

- The pericardial cavity is separated from the peritoneal cavity by the septum transversum.
- The septum transversum and the pleuroperitoneal membranes contribute to major areas of the diaphragm.
- Defects of the diaphragm give rise to congenital herniae in which the abdominal viscera may be pushed into the thoracic cavity.

Chapter 4
The muscular and skeletal systems

The mesenchyme gives rise to the musculoskeletal system. Most of the mesenchyme is derived from the mesodermal cells of the somites and the somatopleuric layer of lateral plate mesoderm (see Chapter 1). The mesenchyme in the head region comes from the neural crest cells. Regardless of their sources, a common feature of mesenchymal cells is their ability to migrate and differentiate into many different cell types, e.g. myocytes, fibroblasts, chondroblasts or osteoblasts. This differentiation often requires interaction with either epithelial cells or the components of the surrounding extracellular matrix.

The skeletal system

The origin of mesenchymal cells forming the skeletal tissues varies in different regions of the body. Mesenchymal cells forming the axial skeleton arise from the mesodermal somites, whereas the bones of the appendicular skeleton are derived from the somatopleuric mesenchyme of the lateral plate mesoderm. After reaching their destination the mesenchymal cells condense and form models of bones. The subsequent differentiation of mesenchymal cells into chondroblasts or osteoblasts is genetically controlled. Various molecular processes, therefore, play a significant role in determining whether mesenchymal cells undergo a membranous ossification or transform into cartilage models, which later become ossified by endochondral ossification.

Development of the axial skeleton

The axial skeleton is composed of the skull, vertebral column, sternum and ribs. This part of the skeleton is derived from the paraxial mesoderm, which is soon organized into the **somites**. The first somites appear on day 20 in the cranial region, and by 30 days approximately 37 pairs are formed. Somites appear as rounded elevations under the surface ectoderm on the dorsal aspect of the embryo from the base of the skull to the tail region. Each somite subdivides into two parts: the **sclerotome** and the **dermomyotome** (Fig. 4.1). The cells of the sclerotome give rise to the vertebrae and ribs, and those of the dermomyotome form muscle and the dermis of the skin.

The vertebral column

The development of the vertebral column passes through three stages. Vertebrae begin as mesenchymal condensations around the notochord, which then transform into

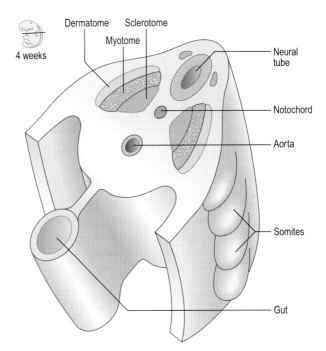

Fig. 4.1 **Differentiating somites in a 4-week embryo.**

cartilaginous models. From the 6th week the ossification of vertebrae begins and usually ends by the 25th year of life.

During the initial mesenchymal stage, the sclerotome cells migrate medially towards the notochord, and meet the sclerotome cells from the other side to form the centrum or vertebral body. Each sclerotome splits into a cranial and a caudal segment (Fig. 4.2A). The cranial half of the sclerotome consists of loosely arranged cells whereas the caudal half contains densely packed cells. The caudal half of a sclerotome fuses with the cranial half of the sclerotome below to form the vertebral body (Fig. 4.2B). From the vertebral body, sclerotome cells move dorsally and surround the developing spinal cord to form the vertebral arch. In each vertebra, the costal and transverse processes develop from the vertebral arches. The vertebral arches of each vertebra join dorsally to form the spinous processes. The formation of the vertebral body is dependent on the inducing substances produced by the notochord and that of the vertebral arch on the interaction of sclerotome cells with the surface ectoderm.

The intervertebral disc has an outer collagenous annulus fibrosus and a central gelatinous core, the nucleus pulposus (Fig. 4.3). The annulus fibrosus develops from the densely packed lower portion of the sclerotome, whereas the nucleus pulposus is derived from the notochord. The rest of the notochord at the level of the vertebral bodies soon disappears.

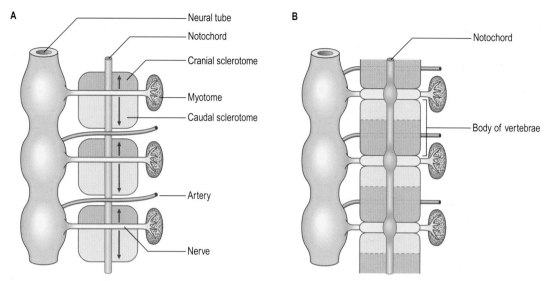

Fig. 4.2 **Diagrams of a 4-week embryo showing the formation of vertebral column from sclerotomes (A, B).** In A the direction of migration of sclerotome cells is indicated by arrows.

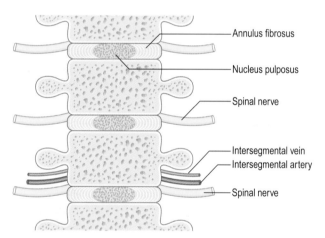

Fig. 4.3 **Adult vertebrae and the position of spinal nerves and intersegmental vessels.**

Because of its formation from two sclerotomes on each side, a vertebra is intersegmental in origin. However, the spinal nerves are segmental as they emerge at the level of the corresponding somite in close relationship to the intervertebral discs.

Clinical box

A **spina bifida occulta** (see Chapter 10 and Fig. 10.5) may occur when the two halves of the vertebral arch fail to fuse behind the spinal cord. This minor anomaly usually occurs in the lumbosacral region, often marked by a patch of hairy skin overlying the affected area, and is seen on routine radiological examination.

The notochordal tissue may persist and give rise to **chordomas**. Most chordomas occur in the midline, most commonly at the base of the skull or in the sacrococcygeal region. These tumours may become malignant, and infiltrate the surrounding bones.

Sternum and ribs

The sternum develops from a pair of cartilaginous bars that form in the ventral body wall. These bars fuse in the midline in a craniocaudal sequence to form the manubrium and the body of the sternum (Fig. 4.4). The anomaly of cleft sternum would occur if the two **sternal bars** fail to unite, and may

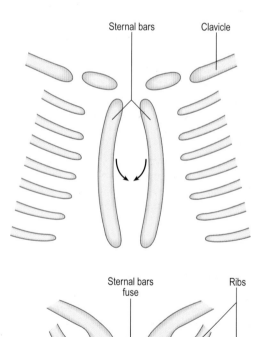

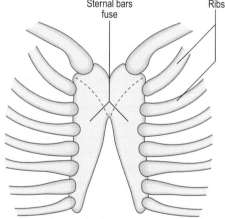

Fig. 4.4 **Development of the sternum and ribs between 42 and 45 days.**

present as a circular defect in the sternum, often an incidental finding at a radiological examination. The ribs arise from the costal processes of the vertebrae in the thoracic region. These become cartilaginous, grow laterally toward the sternum, and become ossified. At other vertebral levels the costal processes do not grow distally but are incorporated into the transverse processes of the vertebrae.

Skull

The skull is composed of the **neurocranium**, which surrounds the brain, and the **viscerocranium**, which surrounds the mouth, pharynx and larynx. Each of these divisions develops by **endochondral** or **intramembranous ossification**. The bones of the neurocranium at the cranial base develop from occipital sclerotomes as three pairs of cartilages, whereas the flat bones of the skull cap develop directly from mesenchyme derived from the neural crest.

The bones of the cranial vault are thin at birth and are separated by fibrous tissue called sutures. The areas where more than two bones meet the unossified mesenchyme are known as **fontanelles** (Fig. 4.5). Six fontanelles are present at birth but the anterior and posterior fontanelles are most prominent. The growth of the brain is accompanied by expansion of skull bones, and both continue to grow during fetal life and early childhood. Not only do the sutures and fontanelles allow skull bones to expand but the fontanelles also override each other during birth to allow the fetal head to pass through the birth canal. Most of the fontanelles disappear during the first year because of growth of surrounding bones, but the anterior fontanelle remains membranous until 18 months after birth.

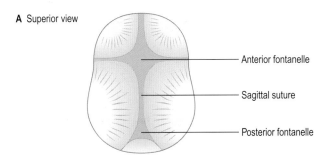
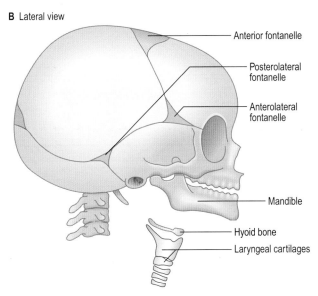

Fig. 4.5 **The fetal skull. (A)** Superior view. **(B)** Lateral view.

The skeleton of the viscerocranium is derived from the first two pharyngeal arches, which support the jaws (see Chapter 11). The mesenchyme in these arches condenses to form a rod of cartilage surrounded by perichondrium. Some of the perichondrium from the pharyngeal arches gives rise to ligaments attached to the skull, and most of the cartilage is replaced by membranous bone. The body and ramus of the mandible develops from the mesenchyme around the ventral end of the first pharyngeal arch cartilage (**Meckel's cartilage**). The condyle and the chin area of the mandible ossify by the process of endochondral ossification. The ear ossicles, the hyoid bone and laryngeal cartilages are also derived from the cartilaginous bars of pharyngeal arches (see Chapter 11).

Development of the appendicular skeleton

The ectodermal cells at the most distal part of the limb bud form the **apical ectodermal ridges**. These ectodermal ridges induce the proliferation and differentiation of the underlying mesoderm, thus forming a rapidly elongating limb precursor. As this growth proceeds the more distal parts differentiate into cartilage and muscle.

The appendicular skeleton consists of the limb girdles and the bones of the limbs. The bones of the appendicular skeleton develop from mesenchymal condensations which become cartilaginous models (Fig. 4.6). The clavicle is the only exception, which begins as a model membranous bone. The centres of ossification first appear in the limb bones during the 8th week. By the 12th week, the shafts of the limb bones are ossified, though the carpal bones of the wrist remain cartilaginous until after birth. The ossification of the three largest tarsal bones of the ankle begins at about 16

A Upper limb 5 weeks

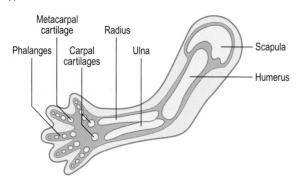

B Lower limb 8 weeks

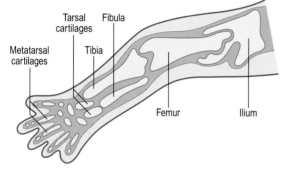

Fig. 4.6 **Developing limb skeleton.** (**A**) Upper limb 5 weeks (**B**) Lower limb 8 weeks.

weeks, but some of the smaller tarsal bones do not ossify until 3 years after birth.

In a typical long bone of a limb, the ossification process begins in the shaft or **diaphysis**, where the cartilage cells enlarge and the extracellular matrix becomes calcified. From this primary centre of ossification, the bone develops towards the ends of the cartilaginous model. A nutrient artery nourishes the central region of the developing bone by penetrating the cartilage. At birth the shafts of long bones are completely ossified, but the ends of the bones or **epiphyses** are still cartilaginous. During the first few years after birth, secondary ossification centres appear in the epiphyses, and bone formation continues in all directions. However, a band of cartilage, the **epiphyseal growth** or

---

cartilaginous plate, remains between the two centres of ossification. The cells of the epiphyseal plate remain active until the long bone ceases to grow, and once the epiphyseal plate becomes ossified to unite with the shaft of the bone, growth is no longer possible. You should refer to an histology textbook for details of histogenesis of bones.

Joints form from the mesenchyme between the developing bones. In a synovial joint, the mesenchymal tissue breaks down to form a cavity, whereas in fibrous and cartilaginous joints, the mesenchyme differentiates into either dense fibrous tissue or cartilage.

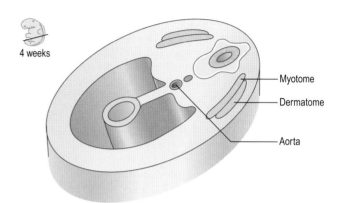

4 weeks

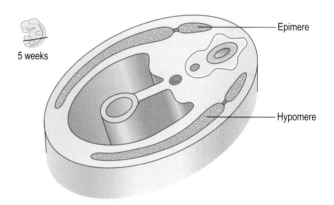

5 weeks

Clinical box

Anomalies of limbs result from a combination of genetic and environmental factors, or teratogenic effects of drugs, or simply mechanical factors. Some deformities involving digits, such as **polydactyly**, **syndactyly** and **lobster claw hand** or **foot**, arise as a result of genetic mutations. Other anomalies, such as **talipes equinovarus** or clubfoot, and **dysplasia of joints**, have been attributed to mechanical compression of the fetus against the uterine wall. **Amniotic bands** also can produce unwanted pressure on developing limbs resulting in constrictions or even complete amputations. This direct pressure on the fetal body may be due to the condition of **oligohydramnios** where the volume of amniotic fluid is too little. Failure of the kidneys to develop may cause oligohydramnios.

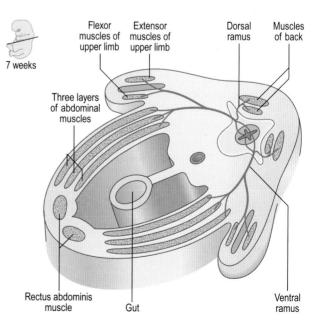

7 weeks

Fig. 4.7 **The origin of the muscular system from myotomes between 4 and 7 weeks showing its innervation.**

The muscular system

Skeletal muscles develop from the **myoblasts** derived from the somites, with the exception of much of the head musculature, which is derived from the pharyngeal arches or the neural crest mesenchyme (see Chapter 11). The muscles of the neck and trunk are derived from the myotomes, whereas the limb musculature develops from myogenic cells that migrate from the ventrolateral region of the dermomyotome of the somite.

Each myotome divides into a dorsal **epimere** and a ventral **hypomere** (Fig. 4.7). The epimere gives rise to the back muscles, including the erector spinae, whereas the hypomere forms the lateral and ventral muscles of the thorax and abdomen. The muscles derived from the hypomere include the intercostal muscles in the thorax, the three layers of the anterior abdominal wall, the rectus abdominis and the infrahyoid muscles. The spinal nerves also divide into dorsal and ventral rami supplying each division of the myotome. The dorsal rami innervate the muscles derived from the epimeres, and the ventral rami innervate the muscles derived from the hypomeres.

The limb muscles differentiate from the myoblasts in the proximal part of the limb bud, and soon receive their innervation from the ventral rami of the spinal nerves. The myoblasts then migrate distally and soon become organized into a dorsal and a ventral muscle mass surrounding the developing skeleton, carrying their innervation with them. Generally, the dorsal muscle mass gives rise to the extensor group of limb muscles and the ventral muscle mass to the flexor group. The ventral rami of spinal nerves, containing sensory and motor fibres, also divide into dorsal and ventral branches to supply the muscles derived from the dorsal and ventral muscle masses respectively. The branches of ventral rami of C5 to T1 form the brachial plexus to innervate the upper limb, and the branches of L4 to S3 form the sacral plexus to supply the lower limb.

During the subsequent development of the lower limb there is a 180° medial rotation compared to the developing upper limb. This accounts for the ventral angle of flexion at the knee contrasting with the elbow where the flexion is dorsal.

Clinical box

Muscles are subjected to considerable variation, but absence of one or more muscles may give rise to functional deficits or **muscular dystrophy**. For example, an infant with abnormal development of the diaphragm may develop breathing problems. Absence of the sternal part of pectoralis major is associated with malformations of the anterior wall of the chest.

Summary box

- The musculoskeletal system is mesenchymal in origin, derived from somites, the lateral plate somatopleuric layer and the neural crest.
- The somites subdivide into two areas: sclerotomes and dermomyotomes.
- The components of the axial skeleton are vertebrae, sternum and ribs. Individual vertebrae develop from sclerotome cells of two adjoining somites.
- The developing skull has two parts: a neurocranium and a viscerocranium. The flat bones of the skull develop in membrane, but the base of the skull is derived from cartilaginous components.
- The limb bones develop from endochondral ossification of cartilaginous precursors. The only exception is the clavicle which ossifies in membrane. The ossification of cartilaginous models of limb bones begins between the 8th and 12th weeks.
- Limb anomalies are multifactorial and form as a result of genetic defects, drug actions and mechanical effects.
- The dorsal muscles of the body wall and trunk are formed from the epimere and the ventral muscles from the hypomere divisions of myotomes. The developmental origins of the muscles are reflected in their innervation by the dorsal and ventral rami of spinal nerves.
- The ventral rami supplying the limb muscles are organized into the brachial and sacral plexuses.

Chapter 5
The respiratory system

Development of the respiratory system

The epithelial component of the respiratory system (including that of the larynx, trachea, bronchi and lungs) develops from the ventral wall of the endodermal lining of the foregut as an outpouching, which grows into the surrounding splanchnopleuric mesoderm as primitive connective tissue surrounding the endodermal **respiratory diverticulum** (Fig. 5.1A). The same splanchnopleuric mesoderm also gives rise to the visceral pleura, cartilage, smooth muscle and the

blood vessels of the lower respiratory tract. The respiratory diverticulum develops at the junction between the cranial and caudal foregut. This diverticulum soon separates from the foregut by the development of bilateral longitudinal ridges, the tracheo-oesophageal folds, that fuse together to form the **tracheo-oesophageal septum**. This septum separates the ventral trachea from the dorsal oesophagus (Fig. 5.1B). Thus, the pharynx communicates with the larynx via the future laryngeal inlet.

The larynx is lined by epithelium derived from the endoderm, whereas the cartilages and muscles of the larynx arise from the **fourth** and **sixth pharyngeal arches** (see Chapter 11).

The lung buds are the paired structures that develop from a single midline outpouching, the respiratory diverticulum (Fig 5.1A). Each lung bud divides many times to form the bronchial tree. The process by which the division of the airways is accomplished is known as **branching morphogenesis** and it is regulated by a variety of molecular signals. There are differences on the two sides: the right lung bud divides into three secondary bronchial buds, forerunners of the three lobes, whereas the left lung bud gives rise to two secondary bronchial buds, to become the two lobes on the left. Thus, a series of rapid further divisions of the airways takes place, penetrating the surrounding splanchnopleuric mesoderm and bulging into the coelomic cavity at the pericardioperitoneal canals (Chapter 3). These two canals are destined to become the right and left pleural cavities, and they lie on either side of the foregut (Fig. 5.2). The pericardial cavity (see Chapter 6) is separated from the primitive pleural cavities by the pleuropericardial folds on each side. The peritoneal cavity is separated from the pleural cavities by the pleuroperitoneal membranes (see Chapter 3). Whilst the splanchnopleuric mesoderm forms the visceral layer of the pleura, the somatopleuric mesoderm lines the thoracic walls and thus forms the somatic layers of the pleura.

Further divisions of the bronchial tree continue but are not completed until after birth. Indeed, full lung maturation is not reached until about 6–7 years of age, and new alveoli continue to be formed up until 10 years of age. Although the earliest stages of the respiratory tract arise in the cervical region of the embryo, as the lungs form they migrate caudally and by the time of birth the tracheal bifurcation lies opposite the 4th thoracic vertebra.

The maturation of the lungs occurs in phases. These different phases are not important other than to appreciate the changes which the lungs undergo. Initially, the lungs are glandular structures histologically, but over time the epithelium thins and tubes or canals form. This is followed by the development of primitive alveoli (Fig. 5.3). Respiration

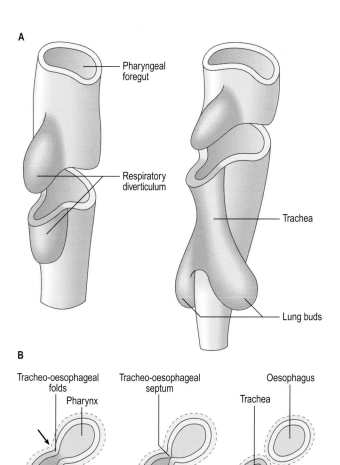

Fig. 5.1 (**A**) The origin of the respiratory diverticulum from the foregut in a 4-week embryo. (**B**) Transverse sections showing the formation of the tracheo-oesophageal septum.

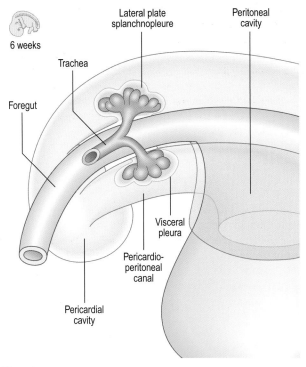

Fig. 5.2 **Lung buds growing into the pericardioperitoneal canals lying on either side of the foregut in a 6-week embryo.**

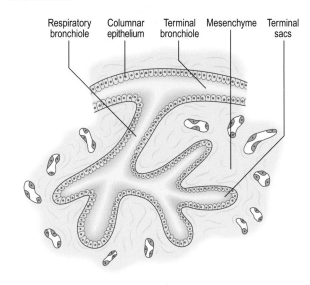

A 25–36 weeks

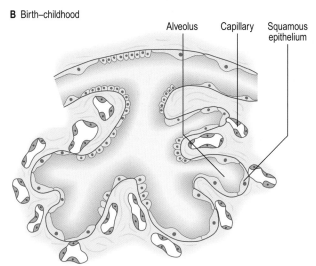

B Birth–childhood

Fig. 5.3 **Histogenesis of the lungs showing thinning of the epithelium and formation of the blood–air barrier. (A)** 25–36 weeks. (**B**) Birth–childhood.

Clinical box

A number of malformations can arise because of incomplete separation of the oesophagus and the trachea (Fig. 5.4). The danger of such malformations in an infant is that swallowed fluids could enter the respiratory tract. The oesophagus can end blindly and not continue with the distal gut tube, leaving a connection with the respiratory tract and the distal gut tube. This is known as a tracheo-oesophageal fistula and is usually associated with **oesophageal atresia**. This leads to abnormal circulation of the amniotic fluid because the fetus normally swallows the fluid and it expels the same volume into its urine. In the presence of a tracheo-oesophageal fistula, the volume of amniotic fluid increases within the amniotic sac, **polyhydramnios**, and an enlarged uterus results. The affected oesophagus may be surgically re-attached to the distal gut tube. These abnormalities arise because of the failure of the tracheo-oesophageal septum to form properly. If the division of the lung buds fails to occur properly the lungs will be smaller than normal, a condition known as **pulmonary hypoplasia**. Unilateral **agenesis** is also possible so that the lung fails to form on one side.

Failure of the type II alveolar cells to produce surfactant results in **respiratory distress syndrome** seen in premature infants. Without surfactant the lungs do not inflate properly, alveoli collapse and respiratory distress results.

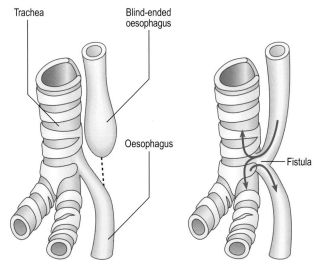

Fig. 5.4 **Types of tracheo-oesophageal fistula.**

is not possible until the cuboidal epithelium of the canals has thinned sufficiently. During this period capillaries come into contact with the thinning epithelial wall and establish the possibility of respiratory gaseous exchange. This begins from about the 7th month. The cells lining the sacs become the alveolar type I cells. Type II surfactant-producing cells appear from about 6 months of age. **Surfactant**, a phospholipid, reduces the surface tension at the air–fluid interface in the alveoli and this helps the air spaces to inflate.

After birth there is a dramatic and rapid change in the lungs to enable air breathing to take place. Prior to birth there is a large volume of fluid in the lungs, which needs to be removed to allow air to pass into the lungs. A number of mechanisms facilitate this process. A large volume of the fluid is removed through absorption by the blood capillaries and lymphatics of the lungs, assisted by the thinning of the epithelium. The pressure of the birth canal itself also helps by squeezing the chest wall to expel fluid.

Summary box

- The respiratory system develops from two germ layers. The epithelial lining arises from the endoderm, which forms the lining of the foregut tube.
- A small diverticulum buds off the ventral surface of the foregut to form the lung bud. This grows into the splanchnopleuric mesoderm, enlarging and bulging into the future pericardioperitoneal canals. These two components of the intra-embryonic coelom become the pleural cavities.
- The lung buds divide rapidly by a process known as branching morphogenesis regulated by a variety of molecular signals. There is, however, an asymmetry in this division such that the left lung has two lobes and the right lung has three.
- The cartilage and smooth muscle of the airways and visceral pleura develop from the surrounding splanchnopleuric mesoderm. The somatopleuric mesoderm lines the future thoracic wall, as parietal pleura.

- Mature alveoli continue to develop until 6 or 7 years of age. Lung development passes though a number of phases: from an initial glandular stage to a tubular phase resulting in formation of the airway tubes.
- After 26 weeks of fetal life the lining of the alveoli thins from a cuboidal to a simple squamous epithelium, thereby facilitating gaseous exchange.
- It is not until after this time that air-breathing is possible, and is a reason why premature infants younger than 26 weeks are often non-viable.
- Type I alveolar cells line the walls of the alveoli; type II alveolar cells produce surfactant, a phospholipid material which reduces the surface tension of the fluid in the lungs. This helps prevent collapse of the alveolar spaces. Infants in whom type II alveolar cells do not produce surfactant may suffer from respiratory distress syndrome.

Chapter 6
The cardiovascular system

One of the first systems to develop in the embryo is the cardiovascular system because of the need to transport oxygen to embryonic cells. In the early embryo, nutrients are derived from trophoblastic digestion of the uterine mucosa, then via diffusion from the contents of the yolk sac. This soon becomes inadequate for the needs of the rapidly growing embryo. As the number of cells in the embryo increase most of the cells lose contact with a surface for diffusion to occur. The initial components of the cardiovascular system appear as **angiogenic cell clusters** in the extra-embryonic mesoderm lining the yolk sac (Fig. 6.1). These give rise to channels that extend into the embryo. The early embryonic blood vessels that appear around the neural plate in a horseshoe-shaped arrangement arise from the unsegmented mesoderm, which forms rostral to the **prochordal plate**. These clusters merge to form the **cardiogenic area** of the embryo, and the cells form tube-like structures, which initially become the **paired heart tubes**. The paired heart tubes bulge into the midline portion of the intra-embryonic coelom, which is the future pericardial cavity. The dorsal aortae develop on either side of the midline and connect with the heart tubes.

Heart tube formation

With the longitudinal and lateral folding of the embryo the heart tubes fuse to form a single tube, which is carried around to the region of the future thorax (Fig. 6.2). The

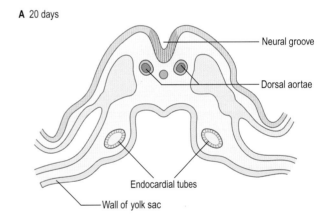

A 20 days

Neural groove

Dorsal aortae

Endocardial tubes

Wall of yolk sac

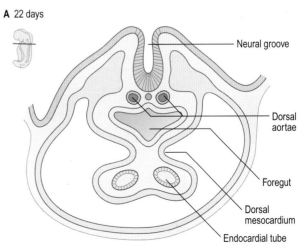

A 22 days

Neural groove

Dorsal aortae

Foregut

Dorsal mesocardium

Endocardial tube

Fig. 6.2 **Transverse sections of embryos at 20 (A) and 22 (B) days showing how the two endocardial tubes come together near the midline as a result of lateral folding.**

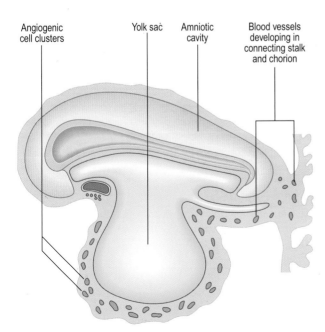

Angiogenic cell clusters

Yolk sac

Amniotic cavity

Blood vessels developing in connecting stalk and chorion

Fig. 6.1 **A longitudinal section of an embryo at about 18 days, showing the formation of extra-embryonic blood vessels.**

heart tube itself comprises an inner endothelial lining and an outer myocardial layer. The outer surface of the heart tube becomes invested in mesodermal tissue, which becomes the future visceral pericardium, or epicardium. This tube is retained within the pericardial cavity by a **dorsal mesocardium** which suspends the tube in much the same way as the gut tube is suspended in the peritoneal cavity. The heart tube is attached at its proximal and distal ends by the future 'great' arterial and venous vessels leaving and entering the heart respectively (Fig. 6.3). Soon, however, the dorsal mesocardium breaks down leaving the heart tube attached merely at the margins of the pericardium. The heart tube itself differentiates during this time, to produce a thicker myocardium.

The heart tube continues to elongate in the pericardial cavity and develops a series of expansions. By day 23 it is too long to be accommodated in the volume available as a straight tube, thus it bends. This forms the **cardiac loop** (Fig. 6.4). The heart tube comprises an atrial portion, which initially is a single chamber, and a ventricular portion: the connection between the two becomes the narrow **atrioventricular canal**. In this region the atrioventricular valves will form later from structures called **endocardial cushions**. These are swellings of mesenchymal tissue, covered by endocardium. The canal connects the common atrium and primitive ventricle. Between the primitive ventricle and the arterial outflow is the **bulbus cordis**, which becomes the right ventricle. The left ventricle arises from the original primitive ventricle. The bends in the heart tube then occur at set places: the **bulboventricular groove** and the **atrioventricular groove**. The bulbus cordis becomes the **conus cordis** that leads from both future ventricles and is the outflow tract which leads on to the **truncus arteriosus** (Fig. 6.4). The truncus arteriosus continues to form the proximal parts of the aorta and pulmonary trunk. The proximal third of the bulbus cordis and the future right ventricle become trabeculated, whereas the conus remains smooth-walled, being associated with the outflow tracts.

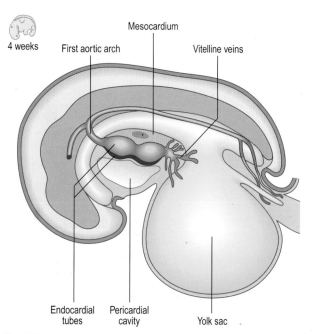

4 weeks First aortic arch | Mesocardium | Vitelline veins

Endocardial tubes | Pericardial cavity | Yolk sac

Fig. 6.3 **The early establishment of the cardiovascular system in a 4-week embryo.**

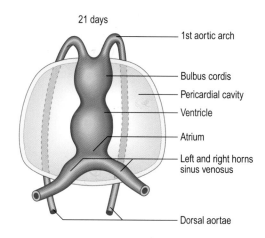

21 days
- 1st aortic arch
- Bulbus cordis
- Pericardial cavity
- Ventricle
- Atrium
- Left and right horns sinus venosus
- Dorsal aortae

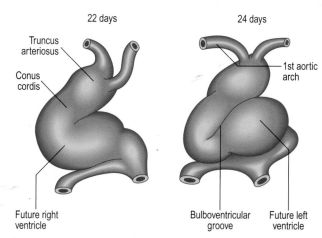

22 days
Truncus arteriosus
Conus cordis
Future right ventricle

24 days
1st aortic arch
Bulboventricular groove | Future left ventricle

Fig. 6.4 **Ventral views of the heart tube (cardiac loop) showing the heart chambers and bending.**

Septation of the heart tube

In the atria, septation begins at about the 4th week. Initially, in the common atrium, a ridge develops in its roof. This is the **septum primum** (or primary septum) and it grows towards the endocardial cushions of the atrioventricular canal (Fig. 6.5). The opening that persists between the septum and the cushion is known as the **ostium primum** (or primary foramen). With further growth the ostium primum is closed, as it reaches the endocardial cushions. Before this closure occurs, however, small holes appear in the septum, which merge to form the **ostium secundum** (secondary foramen) (Fig. 6.5). By this means blood is able to flow between the two atria, an important feature of the fetal circulation (see later). Whilst the septum primum develops another septum begins to form immediately to the right of the septum primum, the **septum secundum** (secondary septum). This grows over the septum primum, but never completely divides the atria, and leaves the opening of the **foramen ovale** (Fig. 6.5). The septum primum filling the foramen becomes the valve of the foramen ovale. This constitutes a vital mechanism to enable circulation of blood from the right side of the heart, which contains oxygenated blood from the placenta, to pass into the systemic circulation, without passing through the pulmonary circulation. The pressure of blood on the right side of the heart is thus sufficiently high to force open the flap valve and allow the blood into the left atrium. After birth, air breathing

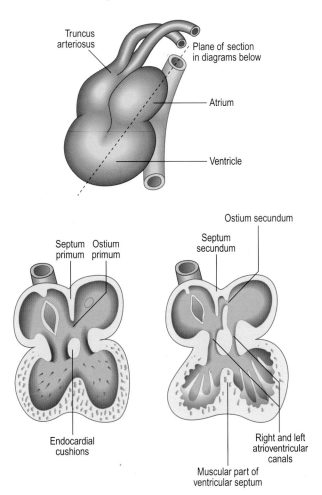

Fig. 6.5 **Partitioning of the common atrium.**

commences and the pulmonary circulation begins, causing pressure to rise on the left side of the heart. The effect of this is to close the flap valve. In most people this results in the formation of a complete septum, the inter-atrial septum. In up to 20% of individuals, however, this is an incomplete seal, and may be opened with a probe, hence **probe patency of the foramen ovale**. Despite this, it is still a functional septum, allowing no passage of blood from the right to the left side. After birth, with the closure of the foramen ovale, the resulting central depression in the interatrial septum is known as the **fossa ovalis**.

Septum formation in the ventricle

The ventricles increase in size and internal volume due to growth of the myocardium. The ventricular wall becomes remodelled, leading to trabeculation. Tissue develops from the floor of the ventricles, midway between the right and left sides, and grows towards the endocardial cushions. This is the muscular component of the interventricular septum (Fig. 6.6). However, it never reaches the cushions, leaving a small gap. This gap is filled by two components: further growth of the endocardial cushions themselves, and downgrowths from the septum that divides the truncus arteriosus (see below). These two components constitute the membranous part of the septum. This part of the septum accommodates the atrioventricular bundle of the conducting system of the heart. Thus, the only myocardial connection between the atria and ventricles is this conducting tissue. This arrangement ensures the sequential contraction of the atria followed by the ventricles, because these two pairs of chambers are otherwise electrically isolated from one another.

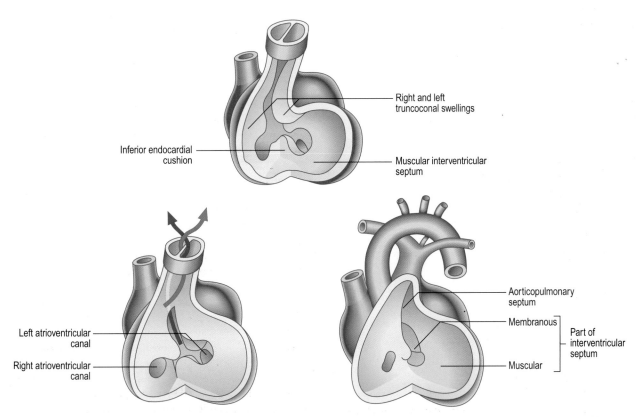

Fig. 6.6 **Partitioning of the ventricles, bulbus cordis and truncus arteriosus between 5 and 7 weeks.**

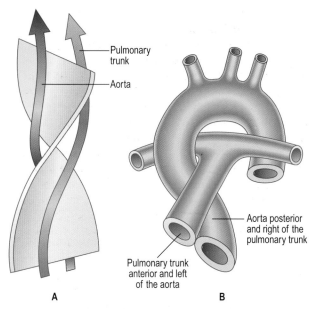

Fig. 6.7 (**A**) The 180° spiralling of the aorticopulmonary septum. (**B**) The adult relationship of the aorta and pulmonary trunk.

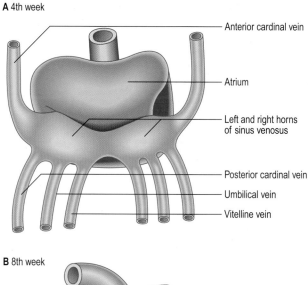

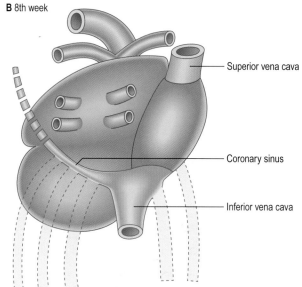

Fig. 6.8 **Posterior view of the heart at 4th week (A) and 8th week (B) showing the fate of the sinus venosus and changes in veins draining into it.**

Septum formation in the outflow tracts of the heart

Initially, the truncus arteriosus is a structure with a single lumen. However, a septum develops dividing the future ascending aorta and the pulmonary trunk. In the 5th week a pair of ridges appear opposite each other within the conus cordis and truncus arteriosus, the **right** and **left truncoconal swellings** (Figs 6.6, 6.7). The two ridges approach one another and form the **aorticopulmonary septum**, and separating the two major outflow tracts of the two ventricles. The septum develops as a spiral structure, which accounts for the spiralling around each other of the pulmonary trunk and ascending aorta (Fig. 6.7).

Development of the venous drainage into the heart

Blood drains into the common atrium via a series of veins. These vessels drain all the blood from the body of the embryo, as well as from the yolk sac and the placenta. It is therefore a complex system, which is initially symmetrical. This system of veins forms the **sinus venosus**. It has right and left sides or **horns**. Initially, each horn empties into the common atrium via a single common opening. Draining into each horn is:

- The **common cardinal veins** into which drain the **anterior and posterior cardinal veins**: by these two veins all the blood from the body of the embryo drains to the atria.
- The **vitelline veins** and the **umbilical veins** which drain blood from the yolk sac and the placenta respectively (Fig. 6.8).

The umbilical veins carry oxygenated blood to the heart and the vitelline veins drain the derivatives of the gut tube. However, the original symmetry of the horns of the sinus venosus is soon lost because of venous blood shunts from the left to the right side of the body. Whereas the right sinus horn becomes the most proximal portion of the inferior and superior venae cavae, the left largely disappears aside from the part that becomes the coronary sinus (Fig. 6.8). As the right sinus horn and venae cavae enlarge, they are gradually drawn into the posterior wall of the atrium. This is the **sinus venarum**, and represents the smooth-walled portion of the atrium, whereas the primitive atrium is displaced anteriorly as a muscular pouch, the right auricle (Fig. 6.9). The smooth and rough parts are separated by a ridge or crest called the **crista terminalis** (corresponding to the **sulcus terminalis**, a groove on the exterior of the heart). From this crest a parallel array of pectinate muscles projects into the auricular portion of the chamber. In the fetal heart the lower part of the crista terminalis forms the valve of the inferior vena cava, and this is arranged so as to direct blood through the foramen ovale into the left atrium. This valve disappears after birth.

The pulmonary veins develop in situ between the lungs and the heart, and enter the left atrium. Gradually, the single opening of the pulmonary vein changes as further parts of

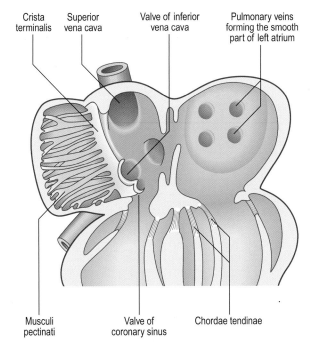

Crista terminalis
Superior vena cava
Valve of inferior vena cava
Pulmonary veins forming the smooth part of left atrium

Musculi pectinati
Valve of coronary sinus
Chordae tendinae

Fig. 6.9 **The interior of the left and right atrium at 8 weeks.**

the two sets of pairs of veins are drawn into the wall of the left atrium: this component forms the smooth-walled component (Fig. 6.9).

Valve formation in the atrioventricular canal and truncus arteriosus

There are two swellings of mesenchyme in the wall of the atrioventricular canal that form the endocardial cushions. These appear at the end of the 4th week at the superior and inferior borders of the atrioventricular canal. Soon after two further swellings arise on the right and left sides of the canal, thus there are four projections into the canal. Subsequent growth causes the superior and inferior cushions to meet and fuse forming right and left atrioventricular canals. The two atrioventricular valves arise from the margins of the atrioventricular canals. Remodelling occurs which results in the formation of the two flap valves. The bicuspid or mitral valve on the left has two leaflets whereas the tricuspid valve on the right has three leaflets. As a consequence of the remodelling, parts of the walls of the ventricles become so thin that the muscular cords connecting the valves with the wall are replaced by connective tissue, the chordae tendinae (Fig. 6.9).

In the truncus arteriosus a similar sequence of swellings of the underlying mesenchymal tissue occurs to form the semilunar valves in the aorta and pulmonary trunk.

Development of the arterial system

The arterial system of the embryo includes the aortic arches and the paired dorsal aortae. These two aortic vessels unite to form the descending aorta which passes the length of the embryo supplying visceral and somatic structures as it does so. The umbilical arteries from the placenta drain the embryo of deoxygenated blood (Fig. 6.10).

Clinical box

The heart tube can loop to the left rather than the right resulting in the anomaly of dextrocardia in which the heart comes to lie on the right hand side of the thorax, not the left. The condition may accompany situs inversus, a condition in which there is a complete mirror-image reversal of the internal organs of the thorax and abdomen. Such a condition is compatible with normal functioning, though there is an increased risk of **volvulus** (see Chapter 7) in the gastrointestinal tract.

Transposition or reversal of the great vessels can occur, and this can result in inadequate oxygenated blood supply to the body. Septal defects constitute a major group of heart anomalies. Ventricular septal defects are the most common heart congenital anomaly. Usually these septal defects arise in the membranous part of the interventricular septum. Atrial septal defects are less common than ventricular septal defects, though ventricular septal defects are often accompanied by interatrial septal defects. Septal defects may result in the 'blue baby' syndrome due to the mixing of oxygenated and deoxygenated blood. A rarer combination of septal and other heart defects is the condition known as Fallot's tetralogy. In addition to the interventricular septal defect there is also hypertrophy of the right ventricular wall, an overriding aorta (that is an aorta that straddles the interventricular wall) and stenosis (narrowing) of the pulmonary infundibulum.

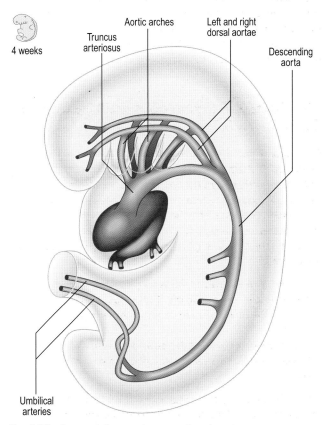

4 weeks
Aortic arches
Truncus arteriosus
Left and right dorsal aortae
Descending aorta
Umbilical arteries

Fig. 6.10 **The arterial system in a 4-week embryo.**

Aortic arches

The outflow channel of the heart is the dilated distal part of the truncus arteriosus, the aortic sac. This sac contributes vessels to the pharyngeal arches that develop in the future neck region of the embryo from about the 4th week onwards. Within each arch the artery develops and meets with the branch from the aortic sac. By this means five/six pairs of **aortic arches** are formed. The aortic arches join the dorsal aorta on each side. Whereas initially there is symmetry in development (Fig 6.11A), changes soon result in an asymmetrical pattern. The aortic sac divides into a right and a left dorsal aorta. The two vessels continue into the body of the embryo where they fuse just inferior to the heart, continuing as a single vessel (Figs 6.10, 6.11A).

The pattern of the subsequent development of the aortic arches is remarkable for two reasons: (1) large portions of the original aortic arches disappear and (2) there are asymmetries for some arch pairs. The 1st pair largely disappear except for the small part that persists as the maxillary artery. The 2nd pair also largely disappear. The 3rd pair form the common carotid arteries, and the external carotid and proximal parts of the internal carotid arteries (Fig. 6.11B). The distal part of the internal carotid arteries form from the dorsal aortae. The fate of the 4th pair is different on the two sides. On the right side the proximal portion of the right subclavian artery forms, whereas on the left side, the 4th arch contributes part of the arch of the aorta. The 5th pair never make any significant appearance. The 6th pair also exhibit asymmetric development. The proximal part of the 6th arch pair form the pulmonary arteries with the pulmonary trunk forming from the truncus arteriosus. On the left side the distal part of the 6th arch persists in fetal life as the **ductus arteriosus**, an important bypass channel for the oxygenated blood from the placenta to avoid passing into the lungs (Fig. 6.11C). Thus, this oxygenated blood passes into the systemic circulation more rapidly than it would otherwise do. On the right side the 6th arch forms the distal portion of the right subclavian artery. The left subclavian artery forms from the 7th intersegmental artery, which is a branch of the dorsal aorta. Along with these changes to the arch pattern, the portion of the dorsal aorta on the right side between the 7th intersegmental artery and the start of the fused dorsal aorta disappears (Fig 6.11B). Whilst these changes take place the position of the heart, and therefore the arches too, alters so that the heart pushes into the future thoracic cavity. Consequently, the carotid and brachiocephalic vessels undergo elongation, and the recurrent laryngeal nerves are similarly lengthened, though their course is different on the two sides. This is because of the different arrangements of the 6th arch pairs. On the left side the nerve hooks under the ductus arteriosus, whereas on the right side the distal part of the 6th arch disappears and hence there is no impediment to the recurrent laryngeal nerve, thus it rides up to hook under the right subclavian artery (Fig. 6.11C).

In the thorax, the descending aorta gives posterolateral intersegmental branches (that lie between adjacent somites) to the thoracic wall (the future intercostal arteries). In the

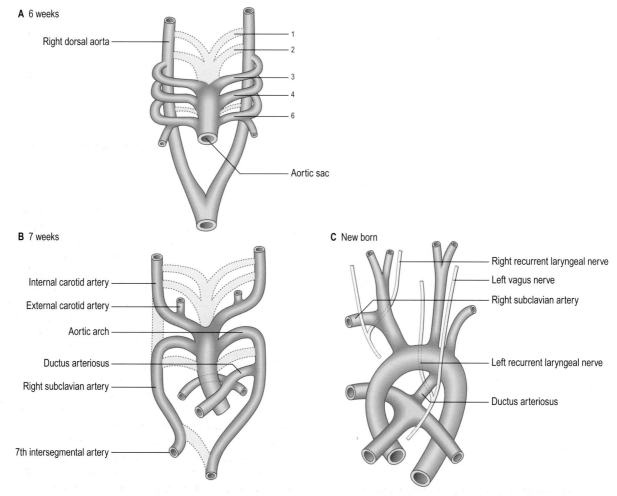

Fig. 6.11 **The aortic arches. (A)** 6 weeks; **(B)** 7 weeks; **(C)** newborn.

abdomen, the descending aorta gives lateral branches to the suprarenal glands, kidneys and gonads, posterolateral intersegmental (lumbar) branches, and ventral branches (celiac, superior mesenteric and inferior mesenteric arteries) to the gut tube.

Umbilical and vitelline arteries

The paired vitelline arteries supply the yolk sac, and the paired umbilical arteries supply the placenta. Both of these sets of vessels undergo considerable changes. The vitelline arteries fuse and form the vessels supplying the foregut, midgut and hindgut, respectively the celiac, superior and inferior mesenteric arteries. The umbilical arteries arise as paired ventral branches of the common iliac arteries (from the dorsal aorta). They conduct deoxygenated blood from the fetus to the placenta where it is re-oxygenated.

Development of the venous system

By the 5th week of development there are three major sets of veins: the vitelline, umbilical and cardinal veins. The vitelline veins drain the gut tube, the umbilical veins bring oxygenated blood from the placenta, and the cardinal veins drain the head and body wall (Fig. 6.12). The proximal portions of both umbilical veins disappear, as does the distal part of the right umbilical vein. The distal left umbilical vein persists and carries the oxygenated blood from the placenta to the liver (Fig. 6.13). Here there is a shunt to avoid much of

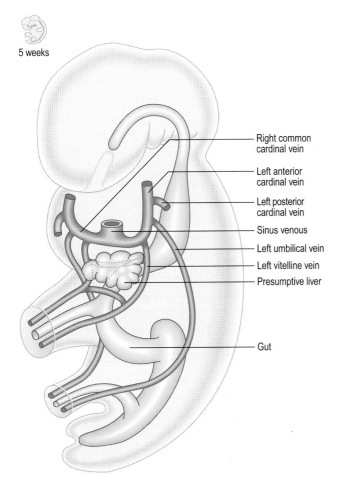

5 weeks

- Right common cardinal vein
- Left anterior cardinal vein
- Left posterior cardinal vein
- Sinus venous
- Left umbilical vein
- Left vitelline vein
- Presumptive liver
- Gut

Fig. 6.12 **The arrangement of the venous system in a 5-week embryo.**

A 6 weeks

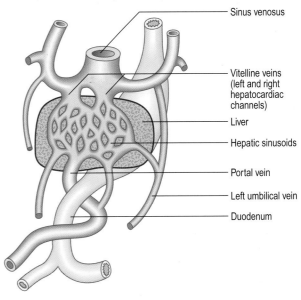

- Sinus venosus
- Vitelline veins (left and right hepatocardiac channels)
- Liver
- Hepatic sinusoids
- Portal vein
- Left umbilical vein
- Duodenum

B 8 weeks

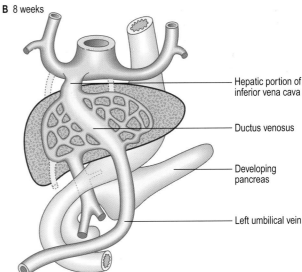

- Hepatic portion of inferior vena cava
- Ductus venosus
- Developing pancreas
- Left umbilical vein

Fig. 6.13 **Fate of the umbilical and vitelline veins. (A)** 6 weeks; **(B)** 8 weeks.

the blood having to enter the liver. The **ductus venosus** passes across the future visceral surface of the liver from the left umbilical vein to the hepatic portion of the inferior vena cava. Also draining into this is the future hepatic portal vein (Fig 6.13A). The fate of the vitelline veins is related to the drainage of the blood from the liver and the fate of the sinus venosus. The growth of the liver interrupts the veins which become incorporated into the liver sinusoids. Blood drains from the liver into the sinus venosus via right and left **hepatocardiac channels**, which also derive from the vitelline veins. The sinus venosus undergoes a left to right shunt so that whereas originally there is an equal volume of blood draining into the sinus via the left and right hepatocardiac channels, the left channel disappears. Thus, all the blood drains via the right channel, and this forms the hepatic portion of the inferior vena cava (Fig. 6.13).

The cardinal veins drain blood from the body wall of the embryo. They do this as anterior and posterior cardinal veins, draining into the sinus venosus at the common cardinal vein. During the 5th week of development additional longitudinal venous channels form in the trunk of the embryo. Initially, these are paired and include the **subcardinal, supracardinal** and **azygos line veins** (Fig. 6.14A,B). Over the next 2 weeks a progressive asymmetry arises resulting in a right-sided dominance. As a consequence some channels enlarge whilst others regress. This changing pattern results in the formation of the inferior vena cava as a single vessel that includes portions of the subcardinal and supracardinal veins. The azygos line veins persist as the azygos system of veins. There is also a left to right shunt in the anterior cardinal veins so that the symmetrical pattern is lost favouring the development of the right and left brachiocephalic veins and their convergence as the superior vena cava. Similarly, at the distal end of the inferior vena cava, the posterior cardinal veins undergo a left to right shunt forming the common iliac veins, draining into the single inferior vena cava. In this way, the left-sided components of the venous system disappear in favour of the right-sided developments, most of which are centred on the formation of the inferior vena cava (Fig. 6.14D).

Changes in the vascular system at birth

Prior to birth the fetus acquires its oxygen via the placenta. To facilitate this process there are a number of differences in the morphology and organization of the vascular system and heart (Fig. 6.15). After birth, with the start of lung breathing, changes occur in the cardiovascular system. The principal change in the heart is the closure of the foramen ovale. This occurs because of the change in pressures in the two atria. Once lung breathing begins blood passes into the pulmonary circulation and hence pressure falls in the right atrium. Coincidentally, pressure rises in the left atrium with the larger volume of blood returning from the lungs. Thus, the septum primum and septum secundum are pressed together causing a functional closure of the foramen ovale that later seals anatomically. The ductus arteriosus is redundant after the start of lung breathing and becomes the **ligamentum arteriosum**. Initially, closure of the ductus arteriosus is stimulated by bradykinin leading to smooth muscle contraction in its wall, and later by replacement of its

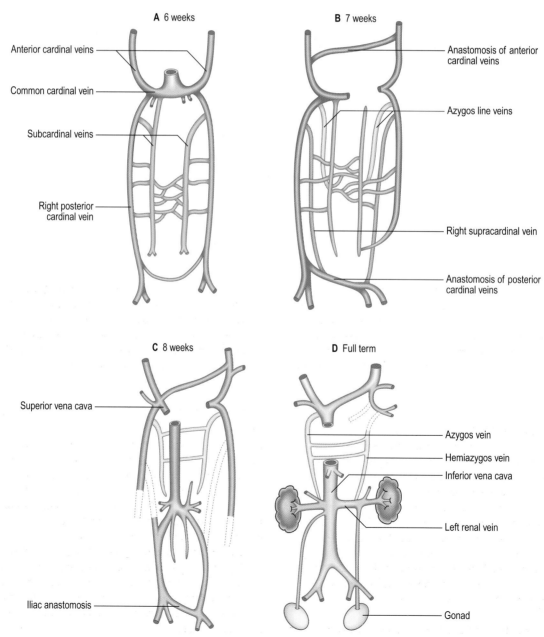

A 6 weeks

Anterior cardinal veins

Common cardinal vein

Subcardinal veins

Right posterior cardinal vein

B 7 weeks

Anastomosis of anterior cardinal veins

Azygos line veins

Right supracardinal vein

Anastomosis of posterior cardinal veins

C 8 weeks

Superior vena cava

Iliac anastomosis

D Full term

Azygos vein

Hemiazygos vein

Inferior vena cava

Left renal vein

Gonad

Fig. 6.14 **The development of the systemic venous system from the cardinal veins.** (**A**) 6 weeks; (**B**) 7 weeks; (**C**) 8 weeks; (**D**) full term.

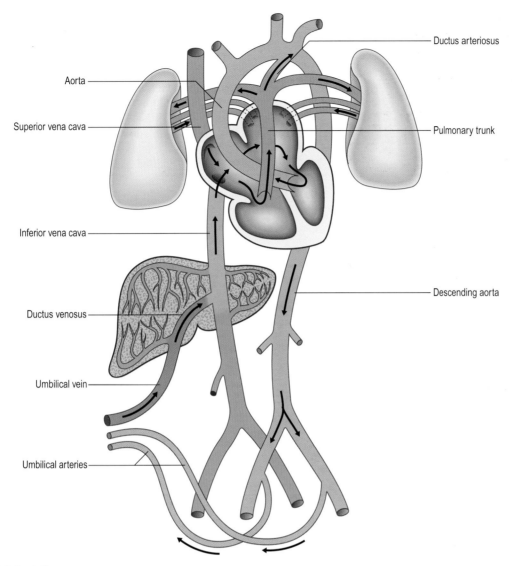

Aorta

Superior vena cava

Inferior vena cava

Ductus venosus

Umbilical vein

Umbilical arteries

Ductus arteriosus

Pulmonary trunk

Descending aorta

Fig. 6.15 **Fetal circulation.**

epithelial lining tissue with fibrous connective tissue. In the fetus the umbilical arteries bring deoxygenated blood back to the placenta. These close after birth, resulting in the formation of the medial umbilical ligaments. The left (and not the right) umbilical vein brings oxygenated blood from the placenta to the fetus. After birth the vein becomes the **ligamentum teres** (**hepatis**), and is found in the free border of the peritoneal ligament, the falciform ligament. The channel responsible for short circuiting the circulation of the liver, the ductus venosus, also degenerates after birth to form the **ligamentum venosum**, and lies in the fissure on the visceral surface of the liver, at the root of the lesser omentum.

Clinical box

There are a large number of potential anomalies of the vascular system, affecting both the arterial and venous systems: one of the most common is the persistence of the ductus arteriosus (often referred to as a PDA, a patent ductus arteriosus). Normally, the ductus closes immediately after birth, forming the ligamentum arteriosum. A PDA reduces the speed with which oxygenated blood can access the systemic circulation. A left to right shunt from between the aorta to the bifurcation of the pulmonary arteries occurs, causing dilatation of pulmonary vessels, breathlessness and ventricular dysfunction.

Often associated with a PDA there may be constriction of the arch of the aorta either just before or just after the junction with the ductus arteriosus: either pre- or post-ductal co-arctation of the aorta. Collateral arterial channels open up to supply the body wall and gastrointestinal tract.

Occasionally, the right dorsal aorta persists resulting in the formation of a double aorta. This may cause compression of the trachea and oesophagus.

Because of the complex symmetrical pattern of vessels leading to the formation of the single inferior vena cava there are a variety of anomalies affecting the venous system, such as a double inferior vena cava, an absent inferior vena cava, a left superior vena cava and a double superior vena cava, for example.

Summary box

- The cardiovascular system is one of the first body systems to develop, in order to carry oxygen and nutrients around the embryo.
- The heart tube develops from unsegmented mesoderm at the rostral end of the embryo, and during longitudinal and lateral folding it is carried round to its future thoracic position, within the future pericardial cavity.
- The tube undergoes septation separating the atria, ventricles and great vessels. Atrial septation involves the development of two septa: the septum primum and the septum secundum. These septa are not complete, enclosing the foramen ovale. This closes at birth as a consequence of the differential pressures on the two sides.
- In the ventricles a muscular upgrowth from the floor of the ventricles plus a membranous component from the endocardial cushions forms the interventricular septum.
- The division of the truncus arteriosus is accomplished by the appearance of the spiral aortico-pulmonary septum, which separates the pulmonary trunk from the ascending aorta. The arterial system develops as two dorsal aortae which fuse after the arch, just caudal to the heart.

- The truncus arteriosus gives rise initially to five/six pairs of aortic arches, which feed into the two dorsal aortae. The symmetry of this pattern is lost as the adult pattern of the arches develops.
- The veins of the embryo drain into the sinus venosus, which also loses its initially symmetric pattern. Draining into the sinus are the umbilical and vitelline veins, draining respectively the placenta and yolk sac. The body of the embryo is drained via the anterior and posterior cardinal veins, via the common cardinal vein into the sinus venosus.
- After birth changes occur in the morphology and organization of the cardiovascular system as a result of lung breathing. Thus, the umbilical arteries become the medial umbilical ligaments, the left umbilical vein (the right disappears) becomes the ligamentum teres hepatis, the ductus venosus becomes the ligamentum venosum and the ductus arteriosum becomes the ligamentum arteriosum. The foramen ovale between the two atria closes leaving the fossa ovalis in the interatrial septum.

Chapter 7
The digestive system

An understanding of the gross anatomy of the gastrointestinal tract is helped by an understanding of the development of the tract. Some of the description below therefore inevitably overlaps with gross anatomy.

The longitudinal and lateral folding (see Chapter 1) of the embryo results in the incorporation of part of the yolk sac. Thus, the endoderm germ layer is incorporated into the embryo and forms the primitive gut tube (Fig. 7.1). In the anterior part of the embryo the incorporation of the endoderm into the head fold results in the formation of the foregut, whilst in the posterior part of the embryo the hindgut forms. The foregut is divided into a cranial and a caudal portion. The cranial portion develops within the head and neck, as the pharynx. This is particularly associated with the pharyngeal arches which are lined by endoderm. In the middle region the midgut forms and initially this is in direct

continuity with the remaining yolk sac. The persisting connection becomes the **vitello-intestinal** (or **vitelline**) **duct**. Each region of the embryonic gut tube is supplied by its specific artery: the celiac, superior mesenteric or the inferior mesenteric arteries for the foregut, midgut and hindgut respectively. In addition to the primitive gut tube, the endoderm layer also gives rise to the parenchyma of the two large glandular organs associated with the gastrointestinal duct, the liver and the pancreas. The connective tissue, smooth muscle and serosal layer of the gut tube and the connective tissue of the pancreas arise from the splanchnopleuric lateral plate mesoderm (see Chapter 1).

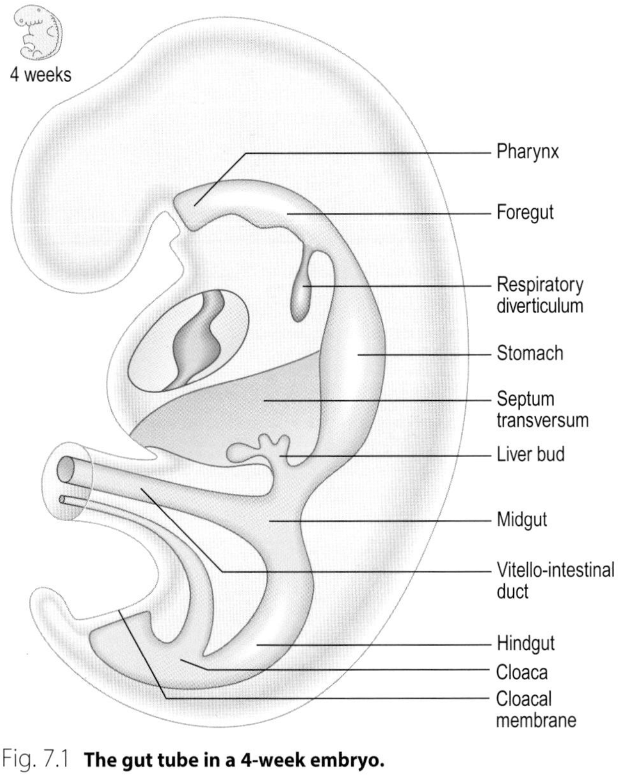

Primitive gut tube

Mesenteries

As the gut tube is incorporated into the body of the embryo it comes to be suspended by a **dorsal mesentery** (Fig. 7.3). This is formed from the serosal membrane derived from the lateral plate splanchnopleuric mesoderm. As the gut tube is incorporated into the body of the embryo 'wings' of amnion push in laterally (responsible for the lateral folding), and these squeeze the connection of the yolk sac and the gut tube. Eventually the endodermal gut tube is formed and it moves ventrally, leaving the overlying splanchnopleuric mesoderm still in contact with the posterior wall of the

4 weeks

Pharynx

Foregut

Respiratory diverticulum

Stomach

Septum transversum

Liver bud

Midgut

Vitello-intestinal duct

Hindgut
Cloaca
Cloacal membrane

Fig. 7.1 **The gut tube in a 4-week embryo.**

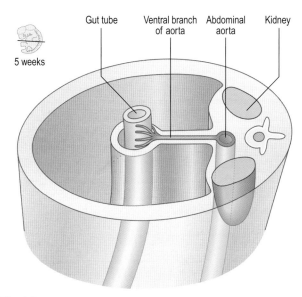

5 weeks

Gut tube   Ventral branch of aorta   Abdominal aorta   Kidney

Fig. 7.2 **A transverse section through the embryo showing the peritoneal and retroperitoneal structures.**

embryo. This suspensory structure is called the dorsal mesentery of the gut tube and extends from the lower part of the oesophagus to the cloacal part of the hindgut. It has two adjacent layers of serosal membrane. The two layers diverge on each side forming the mesentery, which is reflected on to the dorsal wall of the embryo. Since the mesentery is related to the posterior wall of the embryo, close to where the dorsal aorta lies, there is the opportunity for ventral arterial branches of the abdominal aorta to lie between the two layers of the mesentery to gain access to the gut tube without piercing the future peritoneal membrane (Fig. 7.2). In the situation where the gut tube is invested by splanchnopleuric mesoderm all around, aside from the point at which the mesentery begins its investment, the gut tube is said to be intraperitoneal. If an organ is not suspended by a mesentery, thus outside of the peritoneum and in contact with the posterior abdominal wall, it is said to be retroperitoneal, e.g. kidney, parts of the duodenum, pancreas (Fig. 7.2).

With further development the dorsal mesentery is lost for some parts of the adult derivatives of the gut tube: duodenum and the ascending and descending colon. In this situation those parts of the tube are more firmly anchored to the underlying connective tissues. The dorsal mesentery related to the stomach is known as the **dorsal mesogastrium**, and elongates considerably, as the greater omentum.

For the caudal part of the foregut another mesentery develops, the **ventral mesentery**. The ventral mesogastrium is derived from the **septum transversum**, and there is, therefore, a ventral mesentery only for the portion of the gut tube adjacent to the septum transversum. Thus, the terminal part of the oesophagus, the stomach and the initial portion of the duodenum are invested by a ventral mesentery (Fig. 7.3). The liver develops within the ventral mesentery and divides the ventral mesogastrium into two parts. The mesentery lying between the stomach and the liver is the lesser omentum. The part of the mesentery lying between the liver and the ventral wall of the embryo is the falciform ligament. In all these cases the mesenteries are double layers, thus allowing for the possibility of other structures such as blood vessels and nerves to occupy those spaces between the two layers.

Foregut

Development of oesophagus

The initial component of the caudal foregut is the oesophagus. Initially, it too has a dorsal mesentery, which disappears, bringing the oesophagus into its adult position in the posterior mediastinum. As described in Chapter 5 the endodermal **respiratory diverticulum** arises as a ventral bud off the future oesophagus. Because of the growth of the thoracic organs the oesophagus is lengthened.

Development of stomach

At first the stomach is merely a cylindrical tube, like the rest of the gut tube, passing craniocaudally, and it is invested by the dorsal and ventral mesenteries (Fig. 7.4A).
Conventionally, the developing stomach is initially described as being fusiform or flask-shaped. The stomach undergoes a clockwise rotation through about 90° (Fig. 7.4B). The uneven growth is evident by the shorter lesser curvature and the

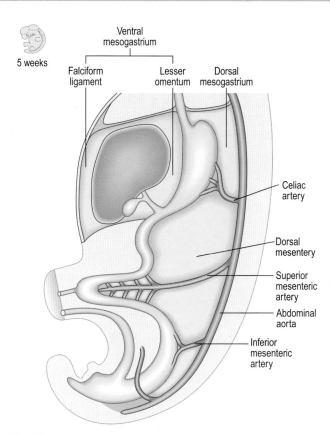

Fig. 7.3 **The dorsal and ventral mesenteries of the gut tube at 5 weeks.**

longer greater curvature of the stomach; this is because the original posterior wall grows quicker than the anterior wall. This rotation of the stomach also results in the dorsal mesogastrium being pulled over to the left side (Fig. 7.5). Consequently, the small compartment lying between the stomach and the dorsal wall of the embryo develops as the lesser sac of the peritoneal cavity (Fig. 7.5). Developing within the dorsal mesogastrium is the spleen, and this is thus carried over to the left side so that it comes to occupy the left hypochondrium in the adult. The portion of the dorsal mesogastrium that lies between the stomach and spleen becomes the gastrosplenic ligament, whilst the part lying between the spleen and the dorsal wall of the embryo becomes the lienorenal ligament (Fig. 7.5).

Lying across the dorsal wall of the embryo is the pancreas (see later). This organ lies so that its left pole is higher than its right. At the point on the dorsal wall of the embryo, where the lienorenal ligament is reflected on to the wall, the tail of the pancreas comes to lie within the double layer of that ligament.

As the liver develops in the ventral mesogastrium and enlarges it is carried towards the right. This accentuates the separate compartmentalization of the lesser sac. The ventral mesogastrium of the foregut is carried rightwards with the liver. The border of the mesogastrium between the liver and the ventral wall of the embryo becomes the falciform ligament. The portion between the stomach and liver becomes the lesser omentum. There is a free border of the lesser omentum (that contains the hepatic artery, bile duct and hepatic portal vein) lying between the duodenum and the visceral surface of the liver (Fig. 7.6).

The lesser sac communicates with the greater sac of the peritoneal cavity (the main part) via the aditus to the lesser

A 5 weeks

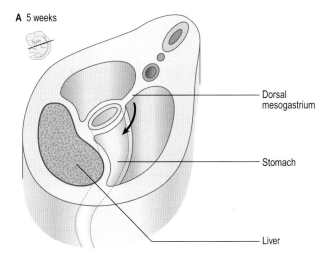
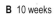

- Dorsal mesogastrium
- Stomach
- Liver

B 10 weeks

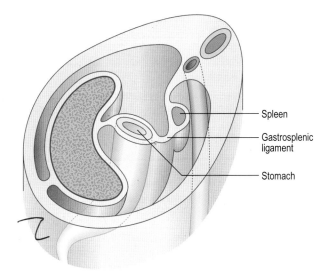

- Spleen
- Gastrosplenic ligament
- Stomach

Fig. 7.4 **Transverse sections through the embryo at the level of the developing stomach showing its rotation.** Arrow indicates the direction of rotation. (**A**) 5 weeks; (**B**) 10 weeks.

10 weeks

Falciform ligament   Lesser omentum   Gastrosplenic ligament

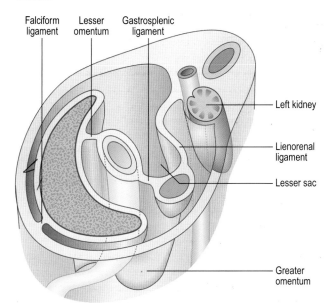

- Left kidney
- Lienorenal ligament
- Lesser sac
- Greater omentum

Fig. 7.5 **Transverse section showing how the mesenteries change during the rotation of the stomach.**

10 weeks

Liver   Lesser sac   Abdominal aorta

Falciform ligament

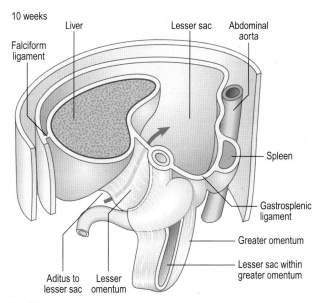

- Spleen
- Gastrosplenic ligament
- Greater omentum
- Lesser sac within greater omentum

Aditus to lesser sac   Lesser omentum

Fig. 7.6 **The formation of the ventral mesogastrium, lesser sac and dorsal mesogastrium at 10 weeks.** The arrow represents the entry point into the lesser sac via the aditus.

sac. The lesser sac itself is limited in its extent by the greater omentum, the latter sealing off each of its lateral borders. In the fetus this means the lesser sac reaches as far as the inferior border of the greater omentum, though the two double layers of the latter gradually fuse, thus limiting the inferior extent of the lesser sac in the adult to a point just beyond the future greater curvature of the stomach (Fig. 7.6).

Development of duodenum

The duodenum arises from two adjacent regions of the gut tube: the foregut and the midgut. The junction between these two regions lies at the mid-point of the duodenum, at the level of the entry of the bile duct (Fig. 7.7). Whereas initially the lumen of the duodenum is hollow, by the 2nd month proliferation of its cellular lining results in a solid duodenum. A process of **recanalization** soon follows so that the hollow lumen is restored. If this process fails then a stenosis of the duodenum results which would cause an intestinal obstruction, and the infant would fail to thrive. As the stomach rotates clockwise the duodenum also rotates to the right, and because of its position comes to lie on the future posterior abdominal wall. This rotation is assisted by the development of the pancreas, which lies within the **mesoduodenum**. As well as the rotation of the duodenum this region of the gut also becomes 'C' shaped resulting from the changes to the stomach, as well as differential growth of the duodenum itself. Because the duodenum arises from both foregut and midgut it has dual arterial blood supplies: branches from the celiac artery (the artery of the foregut)

> **Clinical box**
> In the condition known as congenital hypertrophic pyloric stenosis the smooth muscle of the pylorus is overdeveloped, thereby causing an obstruction. Affected infants exhibit projectile vomiting. The stenosis can be relieved surgically.

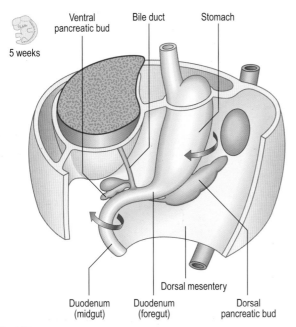

Fig. 7.7 **The development of the duodenum and associated mesenteries in a 5-week embryo.** The arrows indicate the direction of the rotation of the stomach and duodenum.

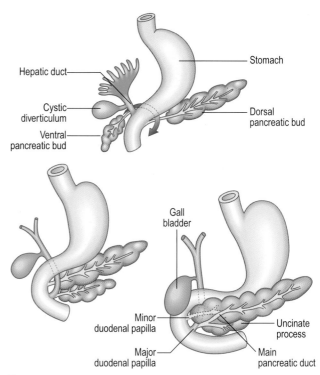

Fig. 7.8 **Development of the pancreas and the duct system between 4 and 6 weeks.**

and branches from the superior mesenteric artery (the artery of the midgut), with corresponding venous drainage to the hepatic portal vein. The stomach is invested on both its anterior and posterior surfaces by peritoneum. The mesoduodenum is lost with further development. Thus, the mesoduodenum is 'plastered' against the abdominal wall, and its posterior layer fuses with the adjacent parietal layer of the abdominal wall. Consequently, the duodenum is covered by peritoneum only on its anterior surface, and this is parietal peritoneum; thus the duodenum is retroperitoneal. This position of the duodenum seals off the lower extent of the aditus to the lesser sac.

Other foregut derivatives

Pancreas
The parenchyma of the pancreas develops from the endodermal lining of the duodenum. **Dorsal** and **ventral pancreatic buds** arise from the duodenum close to the origin of the hepatic bud (see later) from about 4 weeks (Fig. 7.8A). The dorsal bud lies in the dorsal mesentery slightly higher that the ventral bud which lies in the ventral mesentery. However, as the duodenum rotates rightwards the ventral bud moves dorsally. The dorsal bud rotates around the duodenum coming to lie just inferior to the ventral bud (Fig. 7.8B). Thus, the two buds are in contact, both in the same plane, but they enclose the superior mesenteric blood vessels. It therefore appears as though the vessels emerge from within the substance of the pancreas. The two embryological parts of the gland fuse, even though initially the duct systems open separately into the duodenum. Soon, the duct systems fuse too. The duct of the larger dorsal bud becomes the main pancreatic duct, with the duct of the smaller ventral bud merging with that of the dorsal bud. This duct arrangement enters the duodenum at the **major duodenal papilla** in its medial wall (Fig. 7.8C).

Development of liver and biliary tract
The **hepatic diverticulum** arises from the endodermal lining of the foregut just slightly cranial to the opening of the pancreatic duct at about the middle of the 3rd week. This bud of tissue pushes into the septum transversum (see Chapter 3). As this bud enlarges, the connection it has with the duodenum narrows, thus forming the bile duct (Fig. 7.9). The gall bladder develops as a small ventral outpouching, with the connection to the bile duct persisting as the cystic duct. Gall bladder ducts become solid during their early development, but later recanalize. Failure of recanalization results in **extrahepatic biliary atresia**. If this is not correctable surgically, a liver transplant is needed. The hepatic diverticulum enlarges to fill almost all of the septum transversum. The margins of the septum that remain become the peritoneal ligaments that join the liver to surrounding structures, being parts of the ventral mesogastrium. The falciform ligament is reflected from the liver to the ventral wall of the embryo; the triangular and coronary ligaments reflect on to the undersurface of the future diaphragm; and the lesser omentum reflects on to the lesser curvature of the

> ### Clinical box
> Occasionally, the duct from the smaller ventral bud persists and opens separately at the **minor duodenal papilla** (Fig. 7.8C).
>
> Sometimes, the normal direction of rotation of the ventral pancreatic bud around the duodenum is reversed. This anomaly results in a ring of pancreatic tissue around the whole of the duodenum, and this could cause a constriction, or complete obstruction. This is known as **annular pancreas**.

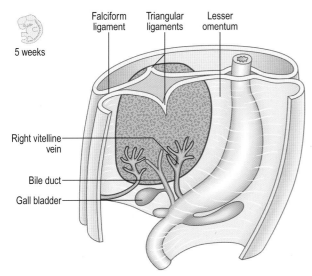

Fig. 7.9 **Formation of the liver from the hepatic bud and the differentiation of the ventral mesogastrium and peritoneal membranes at 5 weeks (coronary ligaments are not shown).**

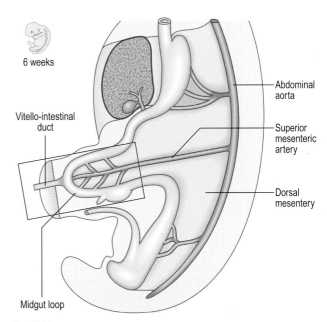

Fig. 7.10 **Herniation of the midgut loop at the end of the 6th week.**

stomach (Fig. 7.9). The future peritoneum covers most of the surface of the liver, with the exception of the bare area, where the organ lies in contact with the diaphragm. The Kupffer cells are bone marrow-derived and invade the liver to line the sinusoids. By the 10th week of development the liver begins to form blood cells, which accounts for the relatively large size of the liver at this stage.

Midgut

Initially, the midgut communicates with the yolk sac via a wide communication, which narrows to become the **vitello-intestinal duct**. The midgut begins at the mid-point of the duodenum, terminating approximately two-thirds of the way along the length of the transverse colon. The artery of the midgut is the superior mesenteric artery, which reaches the gut lying between the two layers of dorsal mesentery. The midgut tube rapidly elongates, which poses a problem in that the peritoneal cavity in which it is contained is too small. As a consequence the midgut herniates out of the abdominal cavity into the umbilical cord at the end of the 6th week (Fig. 7.10). This is the **physiological umbilical hernia**. As the gut tube enters the umbilical cord it rotates anticlockwise approximately 90° (Fig. 7.11A). On return of this loop the tube rotates a further 180° anticlockwise (Fig. 7.11B,C). These rotations take place about the axis of the vitello-intestinal duct/superior mesenteric artery. The increase in space in the abdominal cavity as the embryo grows is thought to account for the reduction of the physiological umbilical hernia. The midgut forms the second half of the duodenum, the jejunum, ileum, ascending colon and two-thirds of the transverse colon. With the rotation of the midgut on return from the hernia, the caecum is carried from its original position under the liver to its adult location in the right iliac fossa (Figs 7.11D, 7.12A). Occasionally, the caecum remains located under the liver (a subhepatic caecum). The vermiform appendix arises at the apex of the caecum.

Most of the midgut retains the original dorsal mesentery, though parts of the duodenum derived from the midgut do

not. The mesentery associated with the ascending colon and descending colon is reabsorbed, bringing these parts of the colon into close contact with the body wall (Fig. 7.12C). The transverse colon retains its dorsal mesentery as the transverse mesocolon, but the latter fuses with the anterior two layers of the greater omentum, thus accounting for the observation that the transverse colon is adherent to the posterior surface of the greater omentum (Fig. 7.12B).

Abnormal physiological herniation of the midgut may be associated with defective body wall closure. There are two main types: **omphalocele** (Fig. 7.13) and **gastrochisis**. In an omphalocele the abdominal viscera herniate through the abdominal wall in the region of the umbilicus, to lie outside the body, though covered with a layer of the amnion. This arises because of incorrect return of the physiological umbilical hernia. In gastrochisis there is a direct herniation of abdominal contents through the abdominal wall into the amniotic sac. In cases of gastrochisis the abnormalities may be correctable, though often with omphalocoele there are other additional abnormalities (often involving the heart) so affected infants are less likely to survive.

The vitello-intestinal duct is normally obliterated but in a small percentage of people it persists as **Meckel's diverticulum**. This pouch is normally located approximately halfway along the length of the midgut in the small intestine. It is significant because it may contain pancreatic or gastric mucosa and the secretions from these tissues can erode the mucosa causing pain, which in its early phase may mimic that of appendicitis. Occasionally, the

> ## Clinical box
> Malrotation of the midgut loop can occur so that rotation occurs clockwise. This can give rise to malpositioning of the intestine, which can cause twisting or **volvulus** of the intestine, and strangulation of the branches of the superior mesentereric artery supplying that portion of the intestine leading to necrosis of the affected part.

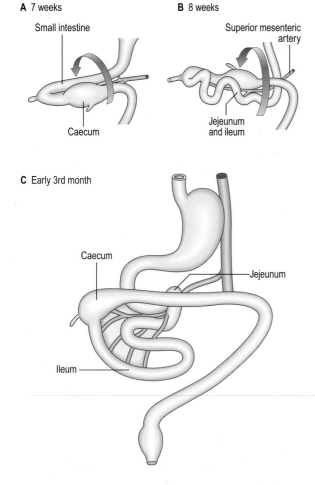

A 7 weeks
Small intestine
Caecum

B 8 weeks
Superior mesenteric artery
Jejeunum and ileum

C Early 3rd month
Caecum
Jejeunum
Ileum

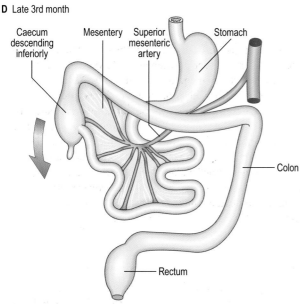

D Late 3rd month
Caecum descending inferiorly
Mesentery
Superior mesenteric artery
Stomach
Colon
Rectum

Fig. 7.11 **Rotation of the midgut loop.** (**A**) 7 weeks; (**B**) 8 weeks; (**C**) early 3rd month; (**D**) late 3rd month. A–C show the 180° anti-clockwise rotation, and (D) the elongation of the midgut loop. The arrow indicates the descent of the caecum.

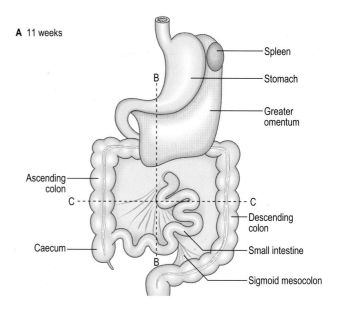

A 11 weeks
Spleen
Stomach
Greater omentum
Ascending colon
Descending colon
Caecum
Small intestine
Sigmoid mesocolon

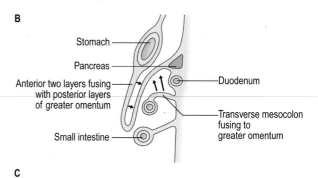

B
Stomach
Pancreas
Anterior two layers fusing with posterior layers of greater omentum
Duodenum
Transverse mesocolon fusing to greater omentum
Small intestine

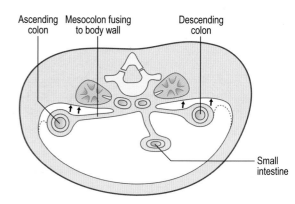

C
Ascending colon
Mesocolon fusing to body wall
Descending colon
Small intestine

Fig. 7.12 **Modification of mesenteries and return of the midgut loop.** Sagittal (**B**) and transverse (**C**) sections at the planes shown in (**A**).

vitello-intestinal duct can persist forming fibrous strands, so-called vitelline ligaments, and these can cause an obstruction to the intestine. The duct may also form a fistula opening on to the anterior abdominal wall. In addition the duct may persist along parts of its course as vitelline cysts. Occasionally the gut tube may become twisted as a volvulus thus causing an obstruction.

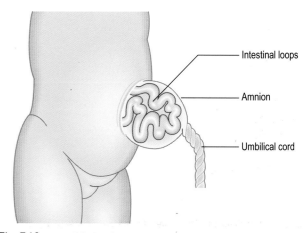

Intestinal loops
Amnion
Umbilical cord

Fig. 7.13 **An omphalocele.**

Hindgut

The hindgut is the region of the gut tube lying between a point approximately two-thirds of the way along the length of the transverse colon to the upper half of the anal canal. In addition, the endodermal layer of the hindgut region forms the epithelial lining of the urinary bladder and urethra. Initially, the hindgut opens into the **primitive cloaca**, which also communicates with the allantois (Fig. 7.14A). A band of mesenchymal tissue (the **urorectal septum**, Fig 7.14A) divides the cloaca into a **urogenital sinus** anteriorly and the rectum posteriorly (Fig. 7.14B, 7.15A). The **allantois** is an unimportant structure in humans functionally. This endodermal tube connects the primitive cloaca to the umbilicus, but it soon becomes a fibrous cord, known as the **urachus**, forming the median umbilical ligament. In some species the allantois contributes to the formation of the placenta. The urorectal septum completes the division of the cloaca when it reaches the **cloacal membrane**, and at that point it forms the perineal body. By this means the future perineum is divided into the anterior **urogenital triangle** and the posterior **anal triangle** (Fig. 7.15A). The anterior part of the cloacal membrane persists until about the 7th week of development when it breaks down, and the anal membrane soon after.

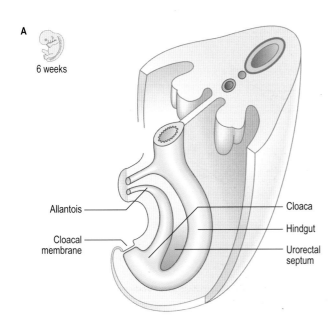

A

6 weeks

Allantois
Cloacal membrane

Cloaca
Hindgut
Urorectal septum

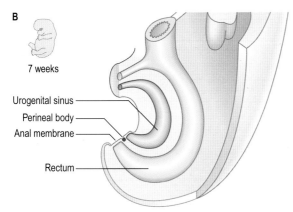

B

7 weeks

Urogenital sinus
Perineal body
Anal membrane

Rectum

Fig. 7.14 **The division of the cloaca by the urorectal septum. (A)** 6 weeks; **(B)** 7 weeks.

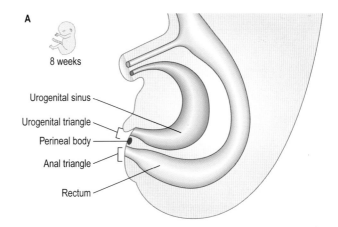

A

8 weeks

Urogenital sinus
Urogenital triangle
Perineal body
Anal triangle
Rectum

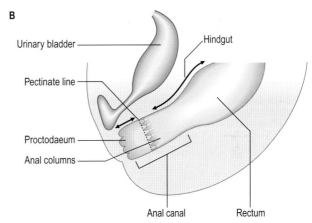

B

Urinary bladder
Pectinate line

Hindgut

Proctodaeum
Anal columns

Anal canal   Rectum

Fig. 7.15 **The subdivisions of the cloaca and formation of the anorectal canal. (A)** 8 weeks; **(B)** newborn.

The mucosa of the upper half of the anal canal is derived from hindgut endoderm, whereas the lower half is derived from the ectoderm, the **proctodaeum** (Fig. 7.15B). At about the end of the 7th week proliferation of the ectoderm occludes the lumen of the anal canal but this recanalizes by the 9th week of development. The pectinate line demarcates the two embryological components of the anal canal. This line is located at the base of the anal columns, and marks a change in the epithelial nature of the lining, as well as the territory of blood and nerve supply, and venous and lymphatic drainage. Thus, the upper half of the anal canal is visceral and the lower half is somatic in origin.

Clinical box

Hirschsprung's disease results if the neural crest fails to develop parasympathetic ganglia in the intestinal wall, thus affecting the motility of the parts of the tract derived from the hindgut region.

If the urachus persists it can give rise to cysts, sinuses or fistulae anywhere along its course from the urinary bladder to the anterior abdominal wall.

A number of misconnections between the components of the cloaca can occur. Fistulae between the terminal part of the hindgut, and the urethra, vagina, or all three, can occur. The anal membrane may fail to break down resulting in an imperforate anus.

Summary box

- The endoderm germ layer contributes the epithelial lining of the gut tube as well as the parenchyma of the liver (and biliary apparatus) and pancreas.
- The gut tube is divided into three regions: the foregut, midgut and hindgut. The foregut comprises cranial and caudal portions: the cranial portion gives rise to the pharynx and is dealt with in Chapter 11. The caudal part becomes the lower part of the oesophagus, stomach and cranial half of the duodenum.
- The midgut endoderm gives rise to the mucosae of the second half of the duodenum, the jejunum, ileum, ascending colon and two-thirds of the transverse colon. It forms a rapidly elongating loop, which results in the formation of the physiological umbilical hernia.
- During this phase the midgut loop rotates in an anticlockwise direction firstly 90° as the loop enters the umbilical cord, and on its return to the abdominal cavity, a further 180°. This takes place between the 6th and 10th weeks.
- The hindgut endoderm gives rise to the mucosae of the rest of the transverse, descending and sigmoid colon, as well as that of the rectum and upper half of the anal canal. It also gives rise to part of the lining of the urinary tract.
- The lower half of the anal canal is derived from an ectodermal ingrowth, the proctodaeum.
- The smooth muscle, connective tissue and visceral peritoneum of the whole of the gut tube is derived from the lateral plate splanchnopleuric mesoderm.

Chapter 8
The urinary system

Morphologically, the urinary and genital or reproductive systems may be considered as one (the urogenital (UG) system) because of their common embryological origins, and because both systems share common ducts. Aside from the germ cells the bulk of the UG system is derived from the intra-embryonic mesoderm. Despite this commonality it is easier to consider the system in its two major functional divisions: the urinary and genital (or reproductive) systems.

Common aspects
The initial structures that develop in the UG system have excretory functions. Subsequently, a number of those structures become adapted for reproductive function, losing their excretory roles. The remaining excretory structures continue to develop as the definitive urinary organs and their associated ducts.

Origins
The UG system originates from the bilateral intermediate cell masses of the intra-embryonic mesoderm (Fig. 8.1). Each cell mass develops craniocaudally in the trunk of the embryo as the **nephrogenic cord** that underlies the **urogenital ridge**, the bulge formed by the underlying differentiating mesenchymal tissue. Cavities appear in the mass at each segmental level, beginning at the most cranial end, which are

primitive kidney tubules. On each side, the most cranial components constitute the **pronephros** and these develop first, then the **mesonephros** develops and finally the **metanephros** appears most caudally (Fig. 8.2). The pronephros is non-functional and temporary, whereas the mesonephros and metanephros produce urine. There is a common pattern for kidney development within vertebrates generally, though the extent to which the pronephros, mesonephros and metanephros subsequently develop varies within different species. The metanephros becomes the definitive human adult kidney.

The urinary system

Two components are necessary for the development of an excretory system: a capillary bed from which the filtration product is derived and a tubule to conduct filtration products to the exterior (Fig. 8.3). The tubule begins as a blind-ended cup-like structure invaginating the capillary bed (or glomerulus) and opens into the exterior (via a convergent series of tubes into the urinary bladder). Thus, there is a **nephric vesicle** (becoming known as either mesonephric or

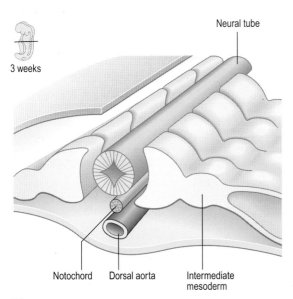

Fig. 8.1 **Transverse section through a 3-week embryo showing the position of the intermediate mesoderm.**

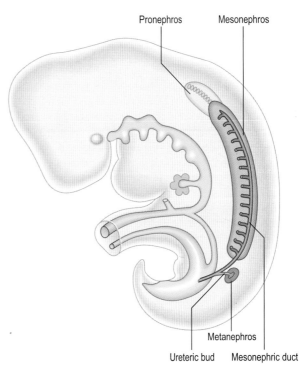

Fig. 8.2 **Lateral view of a 5-week embryo illustrating the three successive kidneys.**

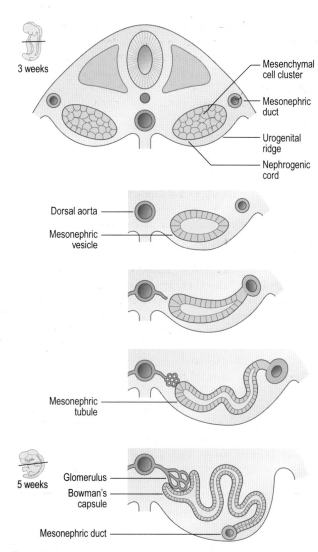

Fig. 8.3 **Transverse sections showing the development of mesonephric tubules between 3 and 5 weeks.**

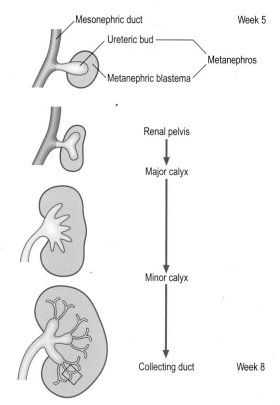

Fig. 8.4 **The development of the metanephros and its duct system between 5 and 8 weeks.** The area enclosed by a box is enlarged in Figure 8.5.

metanephric as differentiation proceeds) and an excretory duct developing from the mesenchymal cells of the intermediate cell mass. The nephric vesicle is the initial part of the tubular system into which the glomerulus invaginates. The tubule opens into the duct (Fig. 8.3) and this pattern occurs at each segmental level. Each tubule lengthens and therefore becomes convoluted, especially so in the metanephros in which the definitive adult nephrons develop.

The pronephros develops at the most cranial end of the nephrogenic cord, but because it is non-functional and is only a short-lived structure in humans it will not be considered further.

The mesonephros begins to develop in the lower thoracic and lumbar segments of the embryo. The cavities, which appear in the mesonephros, become the tubules and connect laterally with the **mesonephric duct**, which also forms from the intermediate mesoderm. The duct lies longitudinally in the embryo draining into the **primitive urogenital sinus**, the future urinary bladder. The urogenital sinus is closed inferiorly by the cloacal membrane (see Chapters 1 and 7), which is derived from the ectoderm and endoderm that lie in contact with each other to form a closure. In some vertebrate species the mesonephros persists as the adult kidney, though not in humans. Parts of the duct system do persist in humans, however, as components of the

reproductive system in the male, as the ductus deferens and the efferent ductules of the testis. In the female the mesonephric duct largely disappears though unimportant remnants may be found between the layers of the broad ligament.

The metanephros (Fig. 8.4) develops at the most caudal end of the nephrogenic cord. The **metanephric diverticulum** or **ureteric bud** arises as an outgrowth from the caudal end of the mesonephric duct. The ureteric bud grows into the nephrogenic cord, the tissue of which condenses around it to form the **metanephric blastema** (Fig. 8.4). The tip of the developing ureter (the ureteric bud) continues to divide to form the collecting ducts and the calyces, each division becoming surrounded by a metanephric blastema. The ureteric bud also forms the definitive adult ureter. The cells in the blastema go on to form the nephrons. These developments are longer and more complex than those of the mesonephros. The blind-ended portion of the tubule, as in the mesonephros, receives an invagination of the glomerular capillaries (Fig. 8.5). The mesonephric duct distal to the ureteric bud is incorporated into the wall of the urinary bladder as the trigone, and also forms the ductus deferens.

The kidneys come to occupy their adult lumbar position later in development, apparently having ascended from their pelvic origin (Fig. 8.6). This is because of the differential growth rates of the abdominal walls and the kidneys, and the regression of the enlarged suprarenal glands.

The metanephric kidney is functional from week 10 and the urine produced at this stage passes into the amniotic fluid. The amniotic fluid is swallowed by the fetus, thus recirculating the water content. However, it is the placenta which removes fetal waste at this stage of development.

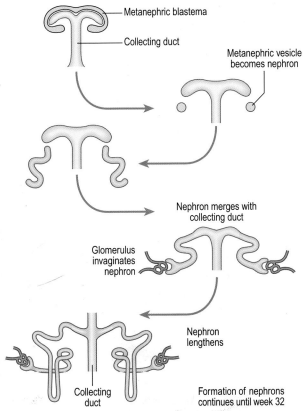

Fig. 8.5 **Successive stages of development of metanephric blastema into nephrons.**

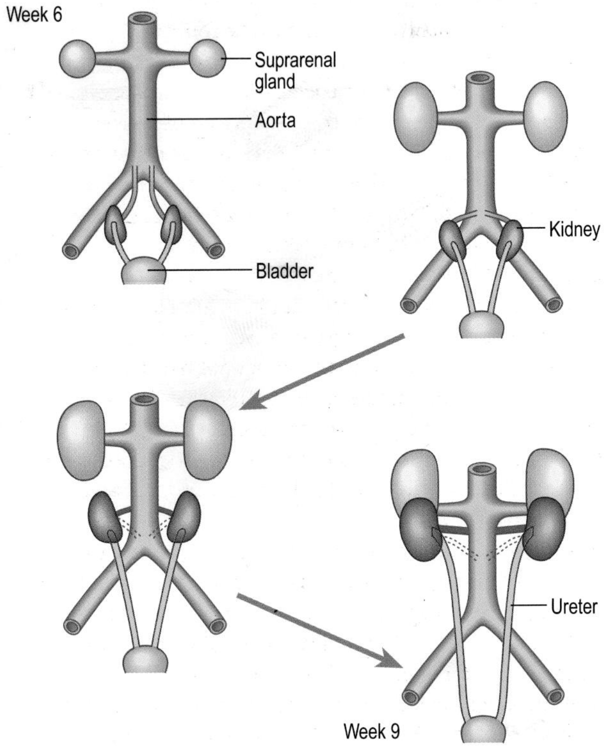

The urinary bladder arises after the cloaca has been divided by the **urorectal septum**. The anterior part is the urogenital sinus, and the posterior component is the anorectal canal (see Chapter 7). Initially the bladder is continuous with the allantois, but the allantois regresses to form the urachus and then the median umbilical ligament after birth.

Clinical box

The developing kidneys are subject to a range of developmental anomalies ranging from **agenesis** to **dysplasia**, or to cyst formation. There are also some possible positional malformations. If the kidneys do not 'ascend' from their pelvic origin then a **pelvic kidney** results. Sometimes both kidneys become so close during their ascent that their lower poles (usually) fuse, a so-called **horseshoe kidney**. This can lead to pressure on the inferior vena cava and oedema of the lower limbs. In cystic, pelvic or horseshoe kidneys, presenting symptoms may include haematuria and recurrent renal infections.

As a consequence of the ascending kidneys a successive series of arterial blood supplies arise from the abdominal aorta. The persistence of an **accessory renal artery** supplying the lower pole of the kidney as well as the renal artery proper is commonly observed.

Summary box

- The UG system is considered as one morphologically because of the common embryological origin and shared elements of the duct systems.
- The bulk of the UG system derives from the intermediate mesoderm.
- The initial structures that develop in the UG system are associated with excretory functions, some of which lose those functions and become adapted for reproductive roles.
- Cavities appear in the intermediate cell mass and differentiation proceeds in a craniocaudal direction, and thus the nephrogenic cord develops along the length of the trunk of the embryo, underlying the urogenital ridges.
- The pronephros, mesonephros and then the metanephros develop from the nephrogenic cord.
- In each embryonic segment an excretory tubule and a nephric vesicle develop from which the urinary tubules arise. The glomerulus is invaginated into the nephric vesicle.
- The metanephroi becomes the definitive adult kidney; the ureteric bud grows out of the caudal end of the mesonephric duct into the nephrogenic cord, thus forming a metanephric blastema.
- Part of the duct of the mesonephros persists as the ductus deferens.
- The metanephro, appear to ascend the posterior abdominal wall to achieve their adult position, as a consequence of differential growth rates.
- From the 10th week the metanephros becomes functional but it is the placenta that removes fetal waste.
- The urinary bladder develops from the urogenital sinus, and is initially continuous with the allantois, the latter regressing to form the urachus and median umbilical ligament after birth.

Fig. 8.6 **The ascent of the kidneys from the sacral to the lumbar position between 6 and 9 weeks.** Note the relatively large size of the suprarenal glands which regress at a later stage.

Chapter 9
The reproductive system

Development of the indifferent gonad

The gonads develop from the intermediate mesoderm that is situated in the paired longitudinal urogenital ridges, the more medial part of these ridges being the **gonadal ridges**. In the 6th week **primordial germ cells** migrate from the wall of the yolk sac via the dorsal mesentery of the hindgut to occupy the gonadal ridges. The arrival of these cells induces the cells in the ridges to form **primitive sex cords** (derived from the mesonephros and overlying coelomic epithelium) (Fig. 9.1A). At this stage the gonad is indifferent or uncommitted (Fig 9.2), and consists of an outer cortex and an inner medulla. During the next week the male and female gonads begin to differentiate (Fig. 9.1B–D). If germ cells fail to migrate to the gonadal ridges the gonads do not develop.

Development of the testis (Fig. 9.3)

The sex-determining gene in the Y chromosome produces a protein (testis-determining factor) that promotes the development of a testis: the primitive sex cords proliferate and penetrate into the medulla to form the testicular cords. Some of those cells differentiate into **Sertoli cells**, whilst the remainder become incorporated into seminiferous tubules. The latter are solid cylinders until after puberty at which time they canalize. The testicular cords anastomose to form the rete testis, which becomes continuous with 15–20 persisting mesonephric tubules, the ductuli efferentes. The testis-determining factor also induces differentiation of gonadal mesenchymal cells into the interstitial **Leydig cells**.

Development of the ovary (Fig. 9.4)

In embryos where no testis-determining factor is produced the primitive sex cords extend into the medulla of the gonad, degenerate and form a vascular stroma resulting in an ovary. The surface epithelium of the female gonad, unlike that of the male, gives rise to second generation cortical cords. In the 4th month these cords invest the primordial germ cells to form the ovarian follicles.

Genital ducts

Initially, two pairs of genital ducts arise in both male and female: the **mesonephric** and **paramesonephric ducts** (Fig. 9.1B, C & D).

In the male, the mesonephric duct loses its urinary function once the mesonephros is superseded by the metanephros. The mesonephric duct becomes the ductus deferens and the epididymis (the main genital ducts in the male), opening into the urogenital sinus (the anterior part of the cloaca) (Fig. 9.1). The secretion of testosterone by the interstitial Leydig cells from week 8 stimulates the mesonephric ducts to differentiate into their adult derivatives. Each seminal vesicle buds out from the distal mesonephric duct. The prostate arises as a bud from the urethra (Fig. 9.5). The regression of the paramesonephric ducts in the male is stimulated by the anti-mullerian hormone, secreted by the Sertoli cells. The old name for the paramesonephric duct was mullerian duct; the old name for the mesonephric duct was wolffian duct.

In the female, the mesonephric duct is not involved in genital duct formation. In the absence of anti-mullerian hormone and testosterone the mesonephric ducts regress in the female. The paramesonephric duct system arises as a pair of longitudinal invaginations (Figs 9.1, 9.2) of the coelomic epithelium that overlies the urogenital ridges. The two ducts lie mainly lateral to the mesonephric ducts, though they cross the mesonephric ducts before entering the urogenital sinus. At their cranial ends the paramesonephric ducts open into the future peritoneal cavity as the future fimbriae of the uterine tubes. The caudal ends of the ducts meet in the midline and fuse to form the **uterovaginal canal**, from which the uterus and upper part of the vagina arises. The canal fuses with the sinuvaginal bulb, a swelling on the urogenital sinus (Fig. 9.6). As the paramesonephric ducts fuse in the midline they bring together two peritoneal folds thus forming the right and left broad ligaments. The upper part of the vagina forms from the fused paramesonephric ducts. The lower part of the vagina arises from the urogenital sinus, from the **sinuvaginal bulb** or later the **vaginal plate**, initially as a solid tube, later canalizing to form the vaginal lumen (Fig. 9.6).

A 5 weeks

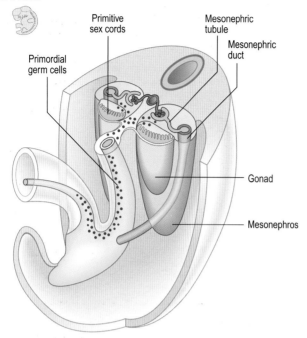

Primordial germ cells

Primitive sex cords

Mesonephric tubule

Mesonephric duct

Gonad

Mesonephros

B **Indifferent stage**–7 weeks

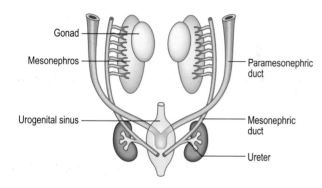

Gonad

Mesonephros

Urogenital sinus

Paramesonephric duct

Mesonephric duct

Ureter

C **Male genital system**–newborn

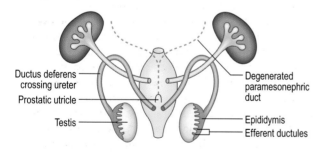

Ductus deferens crossing ureter

Prostatic utricle

Testis

Degenerated paramesonephric duct

Epididymis

Efferent ductules

D **Female genital system**–newborn

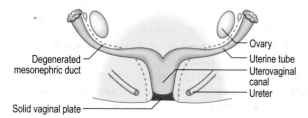

Degenerated mesonephric duct

Solid vaginal plate

Ovary

Uterine tube

Uterovaginal canal

Ureter

Fig. 9.1 **Formation of gonads during the 5th week.** The migration of primordial germ cells to the gonadal ridges is shown in (**A**). (**B**) Indifferent stage at 7 weeks. (**C**) Male genital system in a newborn. (**D**) Female genital system in a newborn.

6 weeks

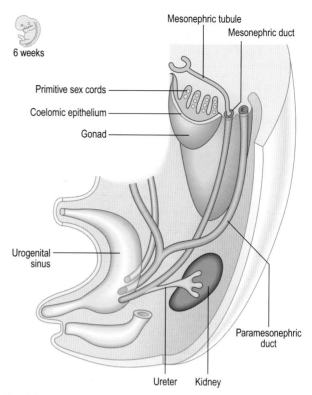

Mesonephric tubule

Mesonephric duct

Primitive sex cords

Coelomic epithelium

Gonad

Urogenital sinus

Paramesonephric duct

Ureter   Kidney

Fig. 9.2 **Indifferent genital system at 6 weeks.**

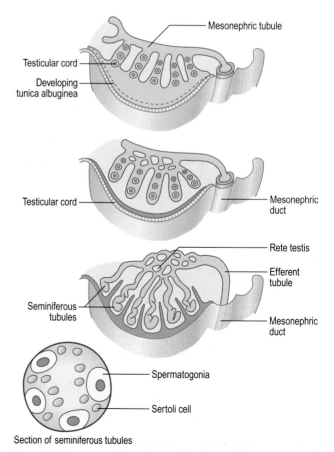

Mesonephric tubule

Testicular cord

Developing tunica albuginea

Testicular cord

Mesonephric duct

Rete testis

Efferent tubule

Seminiferous tubules

Mesonephric duct

Spermatogonia

Sertoli cell

Section of seminiferous tubules

Fig. 9.3 **Development of the testis and male genital ducts.**

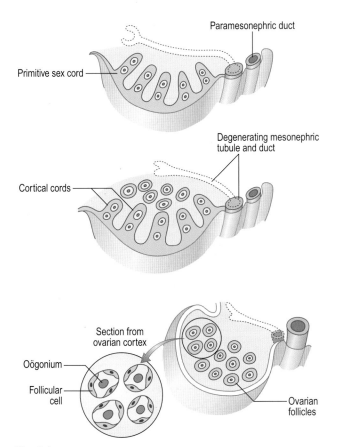

Fig. 9.4 **Differentiation of the indifferent gonad into an ovary.**

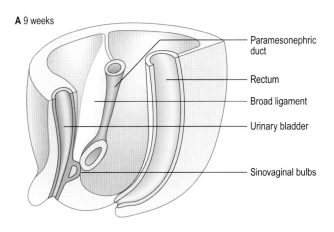

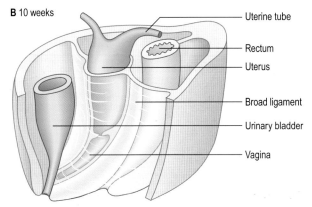

Fig. 9.6 **Formation of the uterus and vagina at 9 weeks (A) and at 10 weeks (B).**

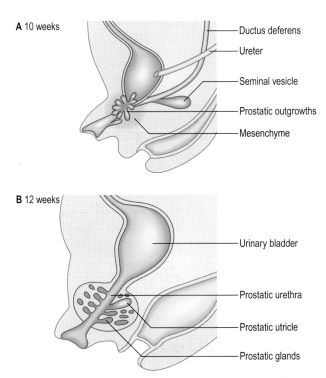

Fig. 9.5 **Development of the accessory glands of the male genital system at 10 weeks (A) and 12 weeks (B).**

Descent of the testis and development of the inguinal canal

In both sexes the descent of the gonad to its adult position is by the guidance of the fibrous strand called the **gubernaculum**. The descent is towards the **labioscrotal swellings** (that form either the labia majora or the scrotum) (Fig. 9.7). In the female the descent of the gonad is as far as the pelvic cavity, on the posterior aspect of the broad ligament. The part of the gubernaculum remaining between the ovary and the uterus is the ovarian ligament; the part between the uterus and the labia is the round ligament of the uterus. Subsequently in the male, an outpouching of the future peritoneum of the coelomic cavity protrudes into the labioscrotal swellings, into the space created by the gubernaculum. This outpouching is known as the **processus vaginalis**, and it precedes the future testis into the scrotum (Fig. 9.7). As the processus vaginalis pushes through the three layers of the abdominal wall it forms the inguinal canal, which is actually a series of slits or apertures in the aponeuroses of the inferomedial parts of the anterolateral abdominal wall musculature.

The testes descend from their initial position high on the future posterior abdominal wall and remain in the vicinity of the deep inguinal rings until about the 7th month of intra-uterine life. The second phase of migration proceeds from then until about the 9th month, and is hormone-dependent.

The factors that are related to the descent of the testis include, firstly, the elongation of the trunk of the fetus, and

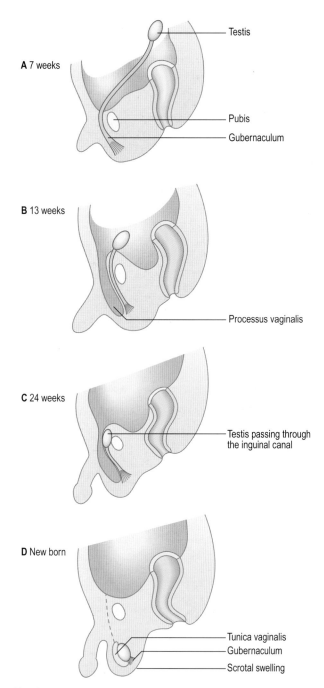

A 7 weeks

- Testis
- Pubis
- Gubernaculum

B 13 weeks

- Processus vaginalis

C 24 weeks

- Testis passing through the inguinal canal

D New born

- Tunica vaginalis
- Gubernaculum
- Scrotal swelling

Fig. 9.7 **Descent of the testis at 7 weeks (A), 13 weeks (B), 24 weeks (C) and in a newborn (D).**

secondly an increase in intra-abdominal pressure arising because of the increasing size of intra-abdominal organs and the regression of the extra-abdominal part of the gubernaculum. As a consequence of the initial development of the testis high on the future posterior abdominal wall, the testis acquires its blood supply from the abdominal aorta, close to the origin of the renal arteries. Thus, the blood supply also migrates inferiorly, resulting in long, thin testicular arteries which pass through the inguinal canals.

External genitalia

At the earliest stages there is no difference in the form of the external genitalia between the two sexes. At the 5th week a

cloacal fold forms on either side of the cloacal membrane and these two folds meet in the midline, anteriorly, as the **genital tubercle**. Subsequently, and lying lateral to the cloacal folds, the **genital swellings** form (Fig. 9.8). The latter give rise to the labia majora in the female or to the scrotum in the male. Thus, the genital swellings fuse in the male but not in the female.

The **urorectal septum** divides the anteriorly placed urogenital sinus from the anorectal canal. In doing so it divides the cloacal membrane into an anterior **urogenital membrane** and a posterior **anal membrane**. The urogenital membrane breaks down and the phallic urethra is therefore in an open groove flanked by the **urethral folds**. The posterior part of the urogenital membrane becomes the anal membrane.

The genital tubercle elongates under hormonal influence to form the penis. The urethral folds are pulled anteriorly to unite by the end of the 3rd month forming the penile urethra. In females, the genital tubercle forms the clitoris, and the urethral folds remain separate to form the labia minora (Fig. 9.8).

> ### Clinical box
> **Uterine duplication and vaginal malformation**
> Failure of the paired paramesonephric ducts to fuse will result in varying degrees of uterine duplication including a **bicornuate uterus** resembling the common non-primate mammalian pattern. Incomplete formation of the sinuvaginal bulbs may result in **vaginal atresia** or duplication.
>
> **Herniae and undescended testes (cryptorchidism)**
> If the processus vaginalis remains in continuity with the peritoneal cavity (normally this connection is lost within the first year of life), then a congenital indirect hernia may develop. If the obliteration of the connection is incomplete with fluid-filled cystic structures remaining these are termed **hydrocoeles**, and may become inflamed or infected. Such structures may occur anywhere along the length of the spermatic cord, or be related to the testes themselves in the layer known as the tunica vaginalis, which is the persisting part of the original processus vaginalis. The abnormalities of the processus vaginalis are shown in Figure 9.9.
>
> **Undescended testes** pose a problem because they are located in the abdomen where the higher temperature is incompatible with normal spermatogenesis. The affected testis may lodge anywhere in the normal path of descent, but this is usually within the inguinal canal.
>
> **Abnormalities of the urethra and urinary bladder**
> Failure of the fusion of the urethral folds results in **hypospadias**, in which the urethra is open on its inferior aspect, either partly or fully. In the much rarer condition **epispadias** the urethral meatus is located on the dorsal surface of the penis. This latter condition is associated with **exstrophy of the urinary bladder**. This is where the interior of the bladder wall is open, due to failure of the closure of the abdominal wall.

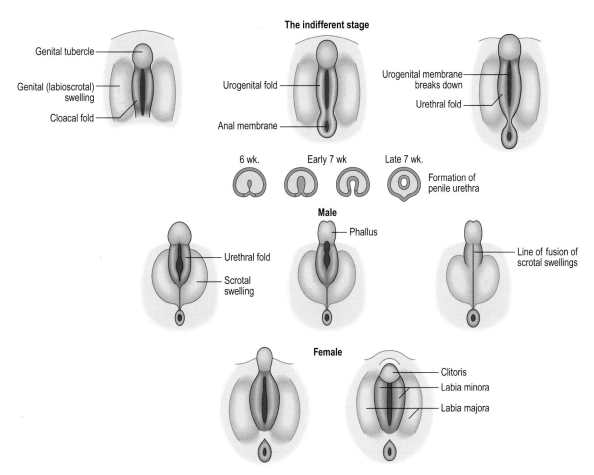

Fig. 9.8 **Formation of external genitalia.**

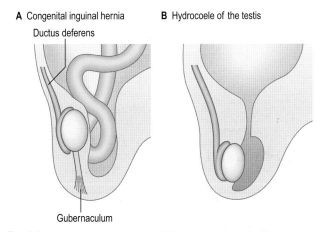

Fig. 9.9 **Abnormal development of the processus vaginalis.**
(**A**) Congenital inguinal hernia. (**B**) Hydrocoele of the testis.

Summary box

- The genital system develops from gonadal ridges which are medial parts of the urogenital ridges.
- Primordial germ cells from the yolk sac migrate into the gonadal ridges in week 6 forming the primitive sex cords.
- A product of the sex-determining gene in the Y chromosome induces formation of a testis; lack of such a protein results in ovary formation.
- Two pairs of genital ducts form initially: the mesonephric and the paramesonephric ducts.
- In the male the mesonephric duct becomes the ductus deferens and epididymis.
- The seminal vesicles bud off the distal mesonephric duct and the prostate buds off the urethra.
- In the female the mesonephric duct almost completely regresses and the uterus, uterine tubes and upper part of the vagina develop from the paramesonephric duct.
- The caudal ends of the paired paramesonephric ducts fuse as the uterovaginal canal.
- The lower part of the vagina arises from the sinuvaginal bulb or vaginal plate, from the urogenital sinus.
- The testes and ovaries descend from their original site to their adult position following the path of the fibrous strand, the gubernaculum.
- The external genitalia begin as cloacal folds in week 5 on either side of the cloacal membrane.
- The urorectal septum fuses with the cloacal membrane to divide it into an anterior urogenital membrane and a posterior anal membrane.
- The cloacal folds meet anteromedially to form the genital tubercle.
- On each side of the cloacal folds genital swellings form which give rise to the labia majora or scrotum.
- The genital tubercle elongates to form the penis in the male, or it forms the clitoris in the female.
- The urethral folds are pulled anteriorly uniting to form the urethra.

Chapter 10
The nervous system

The nervous system forms mainly from the ectoderm layer, at the beginning of the 3rd week (see Chapter 1). The neural plate forms as a thickening which is widest at its cranial end (Fig 10.1A). Laterally, the plate edges thicken to form the **neural folds** (Fig. 10.1B). This is by a process of induction by the underlying notochord and somites. As these neural folds develop they turn towards each other forming the neural groove (Fig. 10.1C), and ultimately fusing as the **neural tube**. The neural tube structure begins in the cervical region and ends caudally. At the cranial end of the tube the brain develops, whereas the remainder of the tube gives rise to the spinal cord. At each end of the tube are the **anterior** and **posterior neuropores** which close in the middle and end of the 4th week respectively (Fig. 10.1D).

The lumen of the neural tube is lined by **neuroepithelial cells** (derived from the neuroectoderm). These cells give rise to the neurons of the grey matter and their processes (dendrites and axons). Some of the axons become invested by myelin and extend into the white matter of the spinal cord. The wall of the neural tube thickens as a consequence of mitosis of the neuroepithelial cells, which become **neuroblasts**. These cells differentiate into mature neurons. The glial cells also differentiate from the neuroepithelial cells once the differentiation of neuroblasts has ended. Whilst the astrocytes and oligodendrocytes arise from the neuroectoderm the microglial cells are bone marrow derived, arising from mesoderm.

In addition to the neuroectoderm cells from which the neurons develop, **neural crest cells** develop on the edges along the length of the neural folds (Fig. 10.1). These cells detach themselves from the edges of the folds lying beneath the surface ectoderm, and migrate laterally to form a variety of structures. The principal derivatives of neural crest cells are:

- dorsal root and cranial nerve ganglia, paravertebral and prevertebral sympathetic ganglia
- parasympathetic ganglia in the gastrointestinal tract
- adrenal medulla cells
- arachnoid and pia mater
- some glial cells, Schwann cells
- dermis in face and neck, and connective tissues and bones in the skull and face
- melanocytes, odontoblasts, 'C' cells of thyroid.

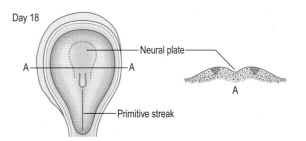
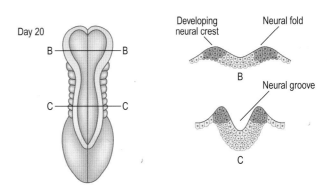
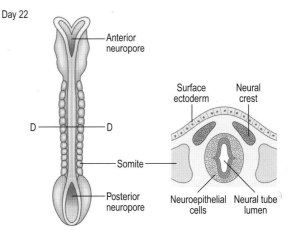

Fig. 10.1 **Folding of the neural plate to form the neural tube between days 18 and 22.** By day 22 the neural tube is detached from the overlying surface ectoderm. Transverse sections through the embryo (**A, B, C** and **D**) are shown in corresponding diagrams on the right.

Development of the spinal cord (Fig. 10.2A,B)

Most of the length of the neural tube gives rise to the spinal cord. As the wall of the tube thickens it comes to consist of three zones. The innermost is the **neuroepithelial (ventricular) layer** and, with the **mantle layer**, it forms the rest of the wall as well as the lining of the central canal

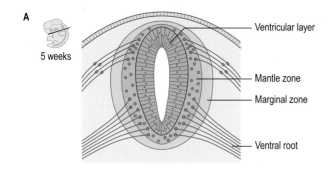

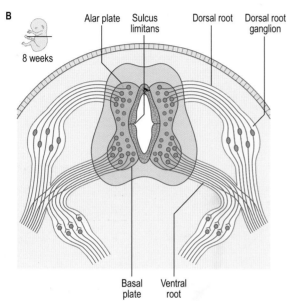

Fig. 10.2 **Development of the spinal cord at 5 weeks (A) and 8 weeks (B).**

through differentiation of the neuroblasts forming thickenings in the dorsal and ventral regions of the cord: the **alar** and **basal plates** (Fig. 10.2B). The alar plate becomes the sensory region (or dorsal horn) of the grey matter and the basal plate becomes the motor region (ventral horn). The lumen of the neural tube in the region of the spinal cord becomes diamond shaped. The pointed dorsal aspect of the tube is the roof plate, whilst the floor plate lies at the opposite pole. Dividing the alar and basal plates is the **sulcus limitans**, a groove. The neurons in the ventral horn give rise to axons that enter the ventral roots. The sensory bipolar neurons in the dorsal root ganglia give rise to axons that enter at the dorsal roots synapsing with perikarya (neuronal cell bodies) in the dorsal horns.

Development of the brain

At the cranial end of the tube three dilations, the **primary brain vesicles** (the **prosencephalon**, the **mesencephalon** and the **rhombencephalon**), develop (Fig. 10.3). They are also known respectively as the **forebrain**, **midbrain** and **hindbrain**. Mainly because of the limited space in which the cranial end of the neural tube is forming there is insufficient space for the lengthening tube. It thus has to bend, and does so in two places: the **cervical** and **cephalic flexures**. The former lies between the rhombencephalon and spinal cord, whereas the latter lies in the region of the mesencephalon (Fig. 10.4B).

The three primary vesicles develop into five **secondary vesicles**. The prosencephalon becomes the **telencephalon** and the **diencephalon**. The telencephalon has bilateral portions which become the two cerebral hemispheres. The diencephalon becomes the thalamus and hypothalamus. The rhombencephalon comprises two regions, separated by the pontine flexure: the **metencephalon** and the **myelencephalon** (Fig. 10.4B). The metencephalon becomes the pons and cerebellum, and the myelencephalon gives rise to the medulla.

The lumen of the neural tube becomes the ventricular system in the region of the brain and brain stem, and the central canal in the spinal cord. The part of the ventricular system lying within the rhombencephalon becomes the 4th ventricle, and that in the diencephalon becomes the 3rd

of ependymal cells (Fig. 10.2A). The neuroepithelial cells in the mantle layer differentiate to become neuroblasts which will eventually be the neurons of the grey matter. The outermost layer of the developing spinal cord becomes the **marginal zone** and contains the axons entering and leaving the mantle zone (Fig. 10.2A). After myelination, this layer looks whitish and constitutes the white matter of the spinal cord. There is further development of the mantle zone

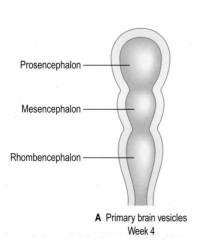

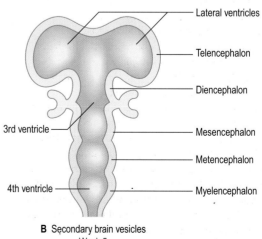

Fig. 10.3 **Development of the brain showing primary brain vesicles at 4th week (A) and secondary vesicles at 5th week.**

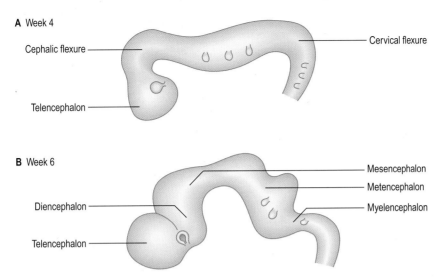

A Week 4

Cephalic flexure

Telencephalon

Cervical flexure

B Week 6

Diencephalon

Telencephalon

Mesencephalon

Metencephalon

Myelencephalon

Fig. 10.4 **The flexures of the brain at weeks 4 (A) and 6 (B).**

ventricle (Fig. 10.3B). The part of the neural tube lumen between the lateral ventricles and the third ventricle is the interventricular foramen and between the 3rd and the 4th ventricle is the cerebral aqueduct, which is continuous with the central canal of the spinal cord.

Until the 3rd month of development the spinal cord extends along the entire length of the vertebral column. Thus, spinal nerves exit at the intervertebral foramen opposite their appropriate segmental level. Subsequently, the vertebral column grows longer than the spinal cord. The spinal nerves, however, still exit at their appropriate intervertebral foramina, thus lengthening accordingly, and forming the cauda equina. The spinal cord ends at about the level of the 2nd lumbar vertebra in the adult.

Clinical box
Neural tube defects

Abnormal closure of the neural tube may occur, especially between the 3rd and 4th weeks, and result in a range of anomalies known as **spina bifida**. This relates to the usual finding of a divided vertebral arch, which is present in all cases of spina bifida. Other changes may involve the underlying neural tube tissue. The clinical problems with spina bifida include problems with lower limb movements, and control of bowel and bladder function. **Spina bifida occulta** is the form where there is a divided vertebral arch, but no other abnormality (Fig. 10.5A). Often in such cases the site of the abnormality is marked by a tuft of hairy skin. In the more serious case of **spina bifida cystica**, neural tissues and their coverings protrude through the vertebral arches and skin, forming cyst-like arrangements. There are two types: **meningocoele**, where the neural tube lies in its normal position, with a cyst formed by the protruding subarachnoid space (Fig. 10.5B), or **meningomyelocoele**, in which the neural tube lies ectopically within the cystic space (Fig. 10.5C). Spina bifida cystica is often associated with hydrocephalus. More rarely, the neural folds do not round up but remain as folds continuous with the surface ectoderm, with no lumen for the neural tube. In this type of spina bifida, the neural tube tissue is exposed and folded, and is known as **rachischisis** (Fig. 10.5D).

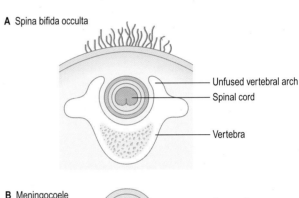

A Spina bifida occulta

Unfused vertebral arch

Spinal cord

Vertebra

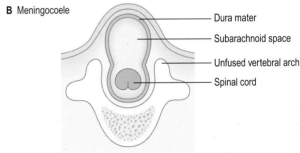

B Meningocoele

Dura mater

Subarachnoid space

Unfused vertebral arch

Spinal cord

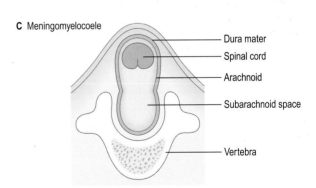

C Meningomyelocoele

Dura mater

Spinal cord

Arachnoid

Subarachnoid space

Vertebra

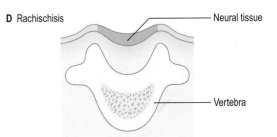

D Rachischisis

Neural tissue

Vertebra

Fig. 10.5 **Various types of spina bifida defects.** (**A**) Spina bifida occulta. (**B**) Meningocoele. (**C**) Meningomyelocoele. (**D**) Rachischisis.

Development of the meninges

The meninges around the cephalic end of the neural tube develop from the neural crest cells, whereas those surrounding the future spinal cord arise from the mesenchyme of the paraxial mesoderm. The dural sac that surrounds the spinal cord ends at the level of the 2nd sacral vertebra.

Formation of the pituitary gland

The pituitary gland develops from two sources: a downgrowth from the floor of the diencephalon (or infundibulum), and an upgrowth from the **stomodaeum** (the ectodermal portion of the oral cavity) known as **Rathke's pouch** (Fig. 10.6). At about the 3rd week Rathke's pouch appears as an evagination growing towards the infundibulum. By 8 weeks the pouch loses its connection with the oral cavity, and lies immediately adjacent to the infundibulum (Fig. 10.6). Thus the pituitary gland has two components: a posterior part derived from the diencephalon

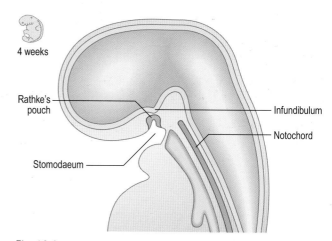

4 weeks

Rathke's pouch

Stomodaeum

Infundibulum

Notochord

Fig. 10.6 **Sagittal section of the cranial part of the embryo at 4 weeks showing development of the pituitary gland.**

with which it is in direct communication, and an anterior part derived from the oral cavity. These two parts are known as the neurohypophysis and the adenohypophysis respectively.

Clinical box

Anomalies of pituitary gland formation

Rarely, a small amount of pituitary tissue from Rathke's pouch develops in the posterior wall of the pharynx, a **pharyngeal hypophysis**. Remnants of Rathke's pouch may give rise to tumours (**craniopharyngiomas**), which are usually benign, though sometimes functional.

Anomalies of cranial development

Anencephaly results from the failure of the cephalic end of the neural tube to close (which then degenerates), and is characterized by failure of parts of the brain to develop normally.

Hydrocephalus is an abnormal accumulation of cerebrospinal fluid in the ventricular system and results from a blockage in the normal drainage pathway for the fluid. This anomaly rarely results in the enlarged head typifying hydrocephalus in the past because of surgical intervention to clear the blockage. The brain and skull tissues may be considerably thinned by this increase in cerebrospinal fluid, though mental impairment is not normally seen.

If the neural tube fails to develop normally in size then the cranial cavity is accordingly smaller. This condition is known as **microcephaly**, and results in mental impairment in many cases.

Chapter 11
Development of the head and neck, the eye and ear

The head region of the vertebrate embryo develops around the cranial end of the neural tube, which expands to form the brain. Inferior to the brain, the face and neck are derived from a series of **branchial** (branchium = gill) arches that lie either side of the stomodaeum (the ectodermal part of the developing oral cavity) and pharynx. In all vertebrates, branchial arches have the same basic plan. In fish and larval amphibians, the branchial apparatus forms a system of gills for exchanging gases between the blood and water. In humans, the branchial arches are called **pharyngeal arches** and they bear some similarities to the gills of lower vertebrates. These arches give rise to the cartilages, bones and muscles involved in chewing and swallowing. The

pharyngeal arches also contribute to the muscles used in facial expression and in speech.

Pharyngeal arches

The pharyngeal arches begin to develop early in the 4th week from **mesenchyme** derived from the neural crest; the lateral plate mesoderm and the paraxial mesoderm also migrate to the head and neck region of the embryo. Five pairs of pharyngeal arches, numbered 1, 2, 3, 4 and 6, form in craniocaudal sequence and by the end of the 5th week, all pharyngeal arches appear as rounded swellings on the surface (Figs 11.1, 11.2). The fifth pharyngeal arch is often rudimentary and soon disappears. Each pharyngeal arch consists of a core of mesenchyme, has an outer covering of

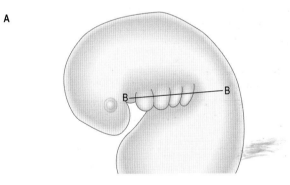

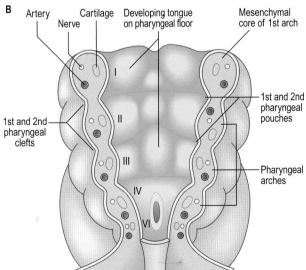

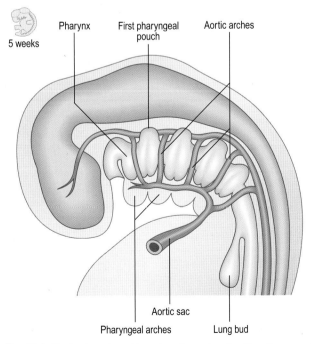

Fig. 11.1 **Sagittal section a 5-week embryo showing the pharyngeal arches.**

Fig. 11.2 **The organization of the pharyngeal arches, pharyngeal pouches and pharyngeal clefts in a 4-week embryo.** Diagram **B** is a horizontal section of the plane shown in diagram **A**.

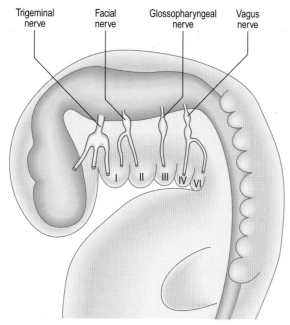

Fig. 11.3 **Sagittal section of a 5-week embryo indicating the cranial nerves supplying the pharyngeal arches.**

their original innervation. Thus, the origin of each muscle can be determined from its nerve supply. The adult derivatives of pharyngeal arch structures, including the cartilages, the muscles and their appropriate cranial nerves, are summarized in Table 11.1. The derivatives of pharyngeal arch arteries are described in Chapter 6.

Pharyngeal clefts

The four pharyngeal clefts separate the pharyngeal arches externally (Fig. 11.4). The first pair of pharyngeal clefts is the only one that contributes to adult structures, namely the external acoustic meatus. The second pharyngeal arch

ectoderm and is lined internally by endoderm. The ectoderm appears as the **pharyngeal clefts** (grooves) between the arches, and the endoderm as the **pharyngeal pouches** (Fig. 11.2B). The first pair of pharyngeal arches not only gives rise to the upper and lower jaw, but they also play a major role in the development of the face and palate.

The mesenchyme in each pharyngeal arch differentiates into a bar of cartilage, the associated muscle and an aortic arch artery (Fig. 11.2B). Each pharyngeal arch also contains a cranial nerve (from nerves V, VII, IX and X) that enters it from the brain stem of the developing brain (Fig. 11.3). The cranial nerves carry the motor fibres to supply the muscles derived from the pharyngeal arches, and also carry the sensory fibres to the developing skin covering them and the mucosal tissue lining them. During further development many pharyngeal arch muscles migrate from their original site of origin to reach their final destination, but they retain

Table 11.1 **Main derivatives of the pharyngeal arches[a]**

Arch	Nerve	Muscles	Cartilage
1st (mandibular)	Trigeminal (CN V)	Muscles of mastication Mylohyoid Anterior belly of digastric Tensor veli palatini Tensor tympani	**Skeletal:** Malleus Incus Spine of sphenoid **Ligaments:** Sphenomandibular ligament
2nd (hyoid)	Facial (CN VII)	Muscles of facial expression Buccinator Stapedius Stylohyoid Posterior belly of digastric	**Skeletal:** Stapes Styloid process Lesser horn and upper part of body of hyoid bone **Ligaments:** Stylohyoid ligament
3rd	Glossopharyngeal (CN IX)	Stylopharyngeus	Greater horn and lower part of body of hyoid bone
4th	Superior laryngeal branch of vagus (CN X)	Pharyngeal muscles Cricothyroid	Thyroid cartilage Cricoid cartilage
6th	Recurrent laryngeal branch of vagus (CN X)	Intrinsic muscles of larynx Striated muscle of oesophagus	Arytenoid cartilage

CN – cranial nerve.
[a] The fifth pharyngeal arch is undeveloped.

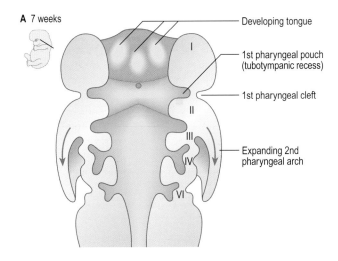

A 7 weeks

- Developing tongue
- 1st pharyngeal pouch (tubotympanic recess)
- 1st pharyngeal cleft
- Expanding 2nd pharyngeal arch

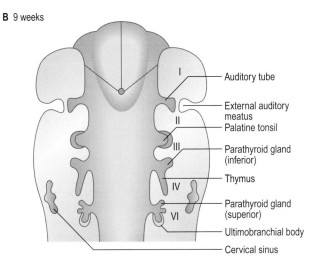

B 9 weeks

- Auditory tube
- External auditory meatus
- Palatine tonsil
- Parathyroid gland (inferior)
- Thymus
- Parathyroid gland (superior)
- Ultimobranchial body
- Cervical sinus

Fig. 11.4 **Horizontal sections of a 7 (A) and 9 week (B) embryo showing the pharyngeal clefts and pharyngeal pouches.**

Table 11.2 **Main derivatives of the pharyngeal pouches**	
Pharyngeal pouch	**Main derivative**
First	Tubotympanic recess, middle ear cavity, auditory tube and tubal tonsil
Second	Palatine tonsil (also pharyngeal and lingual tonsils)
Third	Dorsal: inferior parathyroid glands (parathyroids III)
	Ventral: thymus gland (fuses with the contralateral side)
Fourth	Dorsal: superior parathyroid glands (parathyroids IV)
	Ventral: fuses with ultimobranchial body
Fifth	Ultimobranchial body: fuses with lateral lobes of the thyroid gland; gives rise to the parafollicular cells (C cells) which produce calcitonin

Development of the tongue

In the 4th week, the tongue develops from mesenchymal swellings covered with ectoderm and endoderm on the floor of the pharynx. The three swellings derived from the first arch mesenchyme, the **lateral lingual swellings** and a median **tuberculum impar**, merge with each other to form the anterior two-thirds of the tongue. The second pharyngeal arch makes no contribution to the tongue (Fig. 11.5A,B). Thus, the posterior one-third of the tongue comes from a single swelling, the **hypobranchial eminence**, derived from the third and fourth pharyngeal arches. A V-shaped groove, the **sulcus terminalis**, represents the line of fusion between the epithelium covering the first and third pharyngeal arches (Fig. 11.5C). A midline depression at the apex of the sulcus terminalis, the **foramen caecum**, marks the origin of the thyroid gland (see below).

At first the tongue consists of the pharyngeal mesenchyme, and during the 2nd month muscle tissue migrates into the tongue from the **occipital myotomes**, bringing with it the hypoglossal nerve. The sensory innervation of the tongue reflects the origin of the epithelium covering the pharyngeal arches. Thus the mucosa of the anterior two-thirds of the tongue receives its nerve supply from the lingual branch of the mandibular nerve (nerve of the first arch), and the posterior one-third from the glossopharyngeal and vagus nerves (nerves of the third and fourth arches, respectively). The mucosa covering the vallate papillae, which lies anterior to the sulcus terminalis, is innervated by the glossopharyngeal nerve. This is due to the forward migration of the posterior third of the tongue mucosa across the sulcus terminalis.

The epithelium of the tongue proliferates to give rise to papillae, and the taste buds appear as a result of interaction between the lingual epithelium and the nerve fibres of the facial, glossopharyngeal and vagus nerves. These nerves therefore carry the taste fibres from the mucosa of the tongue. The reason why the chorda tympani branch of the facial nerve innervates the taste buds of the anterior two-thirds of the tongue is explained from studies in comparative anatomy. In vertebrates with gill clefts, the nerves of pharyngeal arches divide to supply the tissues of arches in front of and behind each cleft. Thus, the chorda tympani nerve, the '**pretrematic**' (trema means cleft) branch of the nerve of the second arch, crosses the first pharyngeal cleft and joins the lingual nerve to supply the taste buds in the anterior two-thirds of the tongue, according to the vertebrate pattern.

The taste buds of the vallate papillae are supplied by the glossopharyngeal nerve, despite being in the anterior two-thirds of the tongue.

enlarges and grows rapidly as a flap over the remaining three pharyngeal clefts. This flap contains the platysma muscle and fuses below with the epicardial bulge covering the heart. It is possible that remnants of lower clefts lined with ectoderm may remain beneath the flap forming a **cervical sinus**, but this is normally obliterated (Fig. 11.4B).

Pharyngeal pouches

The endoderm of the pharyngeal part of the foregut grows laterally as pockets on each side of the pharynx. These paired diverticula, the pharyngeal pouches, develop between the arches (Fig. 11.4A). The first pair of pouches, for example, lies in the interval between the first and second pharyngeal arches. The first four pouches are well developed; the fifth is often absent or rudimentary. The ends of the third and fourth pouches each form a dorsal and a ventral part. The first pouch expands into a **tubotympanic recess**; the tympanic (middle ear) cavity and auditory tube are derived from this recess (Fig. 11.4). The tympanic membrane is formed by the ectoderm of the first pharyngeal cleft, an intervening layer of mesenchyme and the endoderm lining the pouch. The derivatives of pharyngeal pouches are shown in Table 11.2 and Figure 11.4.

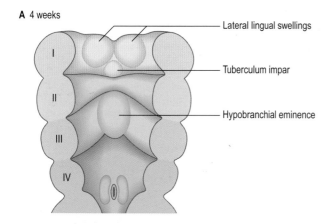

A 4 weeks

- Lateral lingual swellings
- Tuberculum impar
- Hypobranchial eminence

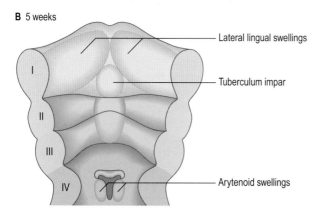

B 5 weeks

- Lateral lingual swellings
- Tuberculum impar
- Arytenoid swellings

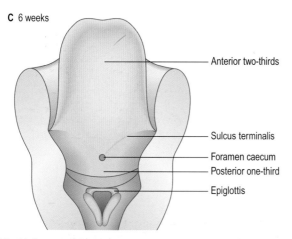

C 6 weeks

- Anterior two-thirds
- Sulcus terminalis
- Foramen caecum
- Posterior one-third
- Epiglottis

Fig 11.5 **Development of the tongue on the pharyngeal floor at 4 weeks, 5 weeks (B) and 6 weeks (C).**

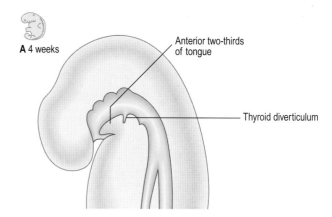

A 4 weeks

- Anterior two-thirds of tongue
- Thyroid diverticulum

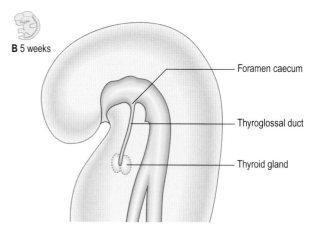

B 5 weeks

- Foramen caecum
- Thyroglossal duct
- Thyroid gland

Fig. 11.6 **Development of the thyroid gland at 4 weeks (A) and 5 weeks (B).**

> ## Clinical box
>
> Thyroid gland abnormalities can occur anywhere along the route taken by the thyroglossal duct. Portions of the duct may fail to degenerate and **ectopic thyroid tissue** can be found in the tongue or the upper neck where the glandular tissue may enlarge as the lingual or the sublingual thyroid gland. Occasionally, a portion of the thyroglossal duct may enlarge as a cyst, which sometimes perforates the skin in the midline of the neck forming a **thyroglossal fistula**.

Development of the thyroid gland

The thyroid gland first appears in the 4th week as an invagination of the endoderm of the floor of the pharynx between the first and second pharyngeal pouches. This point of origin is seen in the adult as the foramen caecum. This soon grows as the **thyroid diverticulum**, descends in the neck, and divides into right and left lobes, connected by an isthmus (Fig. 11.6). The lengthening tube of epithelium between the foramen caecum and the gland is called the **thyroglossal duct**. The thyroid gland becomes detached from the pharyngeal floor when the thyroglossal duct regresses. The lower end of the thyroglossal duct may give rise to a **pyramidal lobe** at the isthmus of the gland, or some smooth muscle, the **levator glandulae thyroideae**.

The developing thyroid gland fuses with the ventral component of the fourth pharyngeal pouch, the **ultimobranchial body**. The parafollicular cells (C cells) of the thyroid, which produce calcitonin, are derived from the cells of the ultimobranchial body.

Development of the face

The face begins to form during the 4th week when the neural crest mesenchyme surrounding the opening of the stomodeum produces five prominences or swellings. These facial prominences consist of a single **frontonasal prominence**, paired **maxillary prominences** and paired **mandibular prominences** (Fig. 11.7A). Table 11.3 shows the structures derived from the three facial **primordia**.

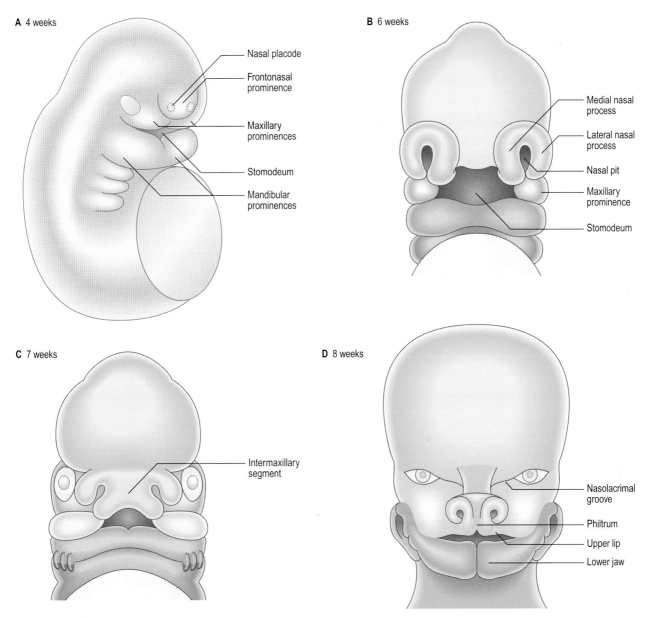

Fig. 11.7 **Development of the face at 4 weeks (A), 6 weeks (B), 7 weeks (C) and 8 weeks (D).**

During the 5th week, two events shape the facial appearance: maxillary prominences enlarge and grow in the medial direction, and bilateral ectodermal thickenings, the **nasal placodes**, appear on the frontonasal prominence. The mesenchyme around each nasal placode forms the **medial and lateral nasal processes** (Fig. 11.7A,B). The medial nasal processes move towards each other, merge in the midline, and form an **intermaxillary segment** (Fig. 11.7C). The maxillary prominences fuse with the lateral nasal process and then with the medial nasal processes to form the upper lip. Each maxillary prominence is separated from the lateral nasal process by a **nasolacrimal groove** (Fig. 11.7D). The ectoderm at the floor of this groove

canalizes to form the **nasolacrimal duct**; its upper end expands to form the lacrimal sac. The maxillary and mandibular prominences merge laterally to form the cheeks and their fusion determines the width of the mouth. The lower jaw is formed when the mandibular prominences merge in the midline (Fig. 11.7D).

Clinical box

Various facial anomalies result from either the failure of the facial prominences to fuse or from variations in the extent to which the mesenchyme in the maxillary and mandibular prominences merges. An **oblique facial cleft** forms when the lateral nasal process fails to fuse with the maxillary prominence, usually resulting in an exposed nasolacrimal duct on the surface. The anomalies **macrostomia**, a large mouth and **microstomia**, a small mouth, are the variations in the mouth opening.

Table 11.3 **Main structures derived from the facial prominences**	
Prominence	**Main structures**
Frontonasal prominence	Forehead, nose, philtrum, primary palate
Maxillary prominences	Part of the cheek, maxilla, zygoma, lateral portion of upper lip, secondary (hard and soft) palate
Mandibular prominences	Lower lip, part of the cheek, mandible

Also during the 5th week, the mesenchyme of the facial structures is invaded by the muscles derived from the pharyngeal arches. The muscles of mastication that develop from the first arch are innervated by the mandibular nerve and the muscles of facial expression derived from the second arch are supplied by the facial nerve.

Development of the nasal cavity and paranasal sinuses

During the development of the face, the nasal placodes invaginate to form the **nasal pits** (see Fig. 11.7B). As a result of the enlargement of the medial and lateral nasal processes on both sides of the nasal pits, the pits deepen and become **nasal sacs** (Fig. 11.8A,B). The nasal sacs grow upwards and are separated from the oral cavity by the **oronasal membrane**, which breaks down during the 7th week to bring the nasal cavities into communication with the oral cavities (Fig. 11.8C). After the formation of the palate, these openings, the **posterior nares**, open into the pharynx. The nasal pits open on the face as the nostrils or **anterior nares**.

During the 9th week, the **nasal septum** develops from the fused medial nasal processes and grows downwards to fuse with the palate. Meanwhile, the **superior**, **middle** and **inferior conchae** form as shelves on the lateral wall of the nasal cavity (Fig. 11.8D). Late in fetal life the maxillary sinuses grow as diverticula from the lateral wall of the nasal cavities into the maxillae bones. The remainder of the paranasal sinuses develop after birth, and their postnatal growth has a significant impact on the shape and size of the face during early childhood and puberty.

Formation of the palate

The palate develops from fusion of the **primary** and **secondary palate** (Fig. 11.9C). The primary palate is derived from the intermaxillary segment and the secondary palate formed by two **palatine processes** or palatal shelves from the maxillary prominences.

Initially each palatine process grows obliquely downwards on each side of the tongue. At the end of the 9th week, the palatine processes elevate rapidly to a horizontal position above the tongue. After they have elevated they then fuse with the primary palate and then with each other from anterior to posterior joining in the midline (Fig. 11.9A,B) at the palatine raphe. At the same time, the frontonasal process and the medial nasal processes form the nasal septum; the latter grows down to meet the upper surface of the palate.

The palatine processes elevate very rapidly, over minutes or hours. Their mechanical elevation and fusion are aided by the accumulation of hyaluronic acid and the alignment of collagen fibrils within the palatine process mesenchyme. The hyaluronic acid causes swelling and expansion of the palatine processes, and the collagen fibrils orientate in a horizontal plane. During week 9, the tongue muscles also become functional, thus creating space for the palatine shelves to elevate.

A 6 weeks

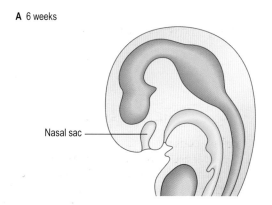

Nasal sac

B 6.5 weeks

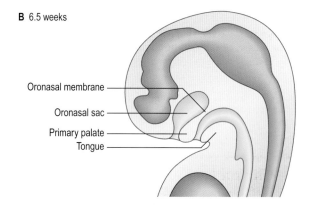

Oronasal membrane
Oronasal sac
Primary palate
Tongue

C 7 weeks

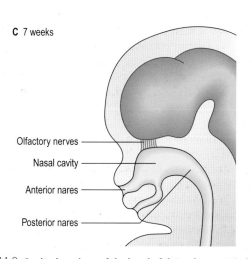

Olfactory nerves
Nasal cavity
Anterior nares
Posterior nares

D 12 weeks

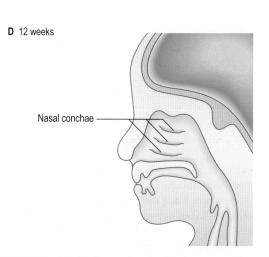

Nasal conchae

Fig. 11.8 **Sagittal sections of the head of the embryo at weeks 6 (A), 6.5 (B), 7 (C) and 12 (D) illustrating the development of the nasal cavities.**

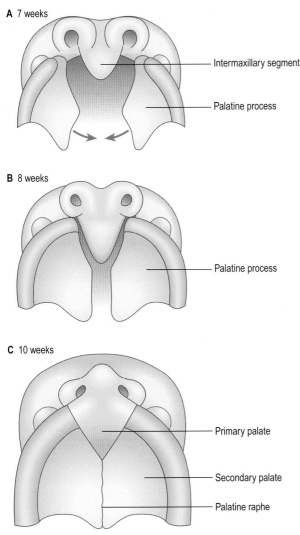

Fig. 11.9 **Diagrams illustrating the formation of the palate as seen from below at 7 weeks (A); 8 weeks (B) and 10 weeks (C).**

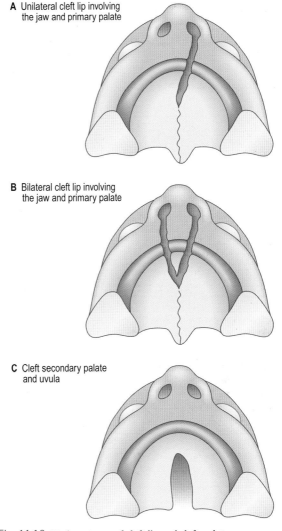

Fig. 11.10 **Various types of cleft lip and cleft palate.**

Clinical box

Cleft lip and **cleft palate** are common defects that result in abnormal facial appearance, defective speech and trouble with feeding. The cleft palate results when the two palatal shelves fail to meet and fuse with each other. There are two major groups of cleft lip and palate, anterior and posterior deformities, with the incisive foramen as the dividing landmark. The anterior deformities include cleft lip, with or without cleft upper jaw, and cleft between the primary and secondary palates (Fig. 11.10A,B). Those that lie posterior to the incisive foramen include cleft secondary palate and cleft uvula (Fig. 11.10C).

Any component of palatal development could cause cleft palate: insufficient mesenchyme or matrix for shelf elevation, shelf elevation being too late, or incomplete fusion. Certain drugs taken during pregnancy will increase the incidence of cleft palate. These abnormalities can be very successfully corrected by surgery after birth.

Development of the eye and ear

Ectodermal placodes

The two paired sense organs, the eyes and the ears, arise from **ectodermal placodes** in the head region of the embryo. Placodes are thickened areas of ectoderm, which form as a result of interaction between the neural tube and overlying ectoderm. The placode cells become columnar, invaginate, and migrate deep to the surface ectoderm. The placodes in the cranial region contribute to the sense organs such as the olfactory epithelium, the internal ear and the lens of the eye. The placodes associated with the pharyngeal arches give rise to the sensory ganglia of the cranial nerves.

The eye

The earliest indication of the eye is in the form of the **optic vesicle**, which develops at the beginning of the 4th week as an outgrowth from the lateral wall of the forebrain. The optic vesicle acts on the surface ectoderm to induce the development of the **lens placode** (Fig. 11.11A). Simultaneously, the connection between the optic vesicle and the brain narrows to form the **optic stalk**. The lens placode invaginates to form the lens vesicle, which soon detaches from the surface ectoderm and sinks into the optic

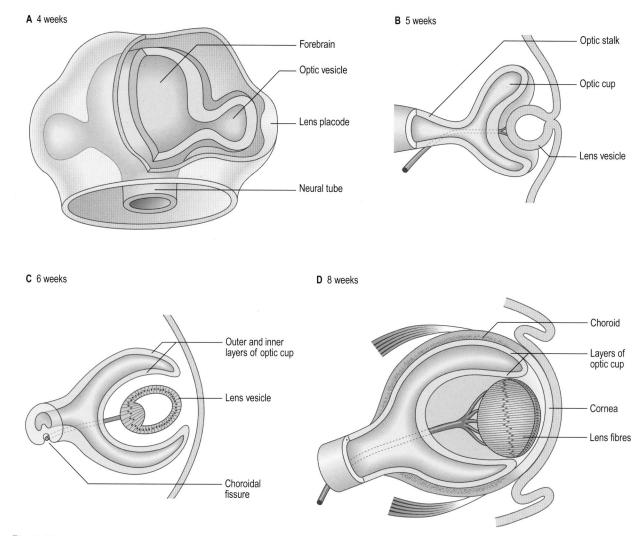

A 4 weeks
- Forebrain
- Optic vesicle
- Lens placode
- Neural tube

B 5 weeks
- Optic stalk
- Optic cup
- Lens vesicle

C 6 weeks
- Outer and inner layers of optic cup
- Lens vesicle
- Choroidal fissure

D 8 weeks
- Choroid
- Layers of optic cup
- Cornea
- Lens fibres

Fig 11.11 **Development of the eye at 4 weeks (A); 5 weeks (B) 6 weeks (C) and 8 weeks (D).**

vesicle (Fig. 11.11A). The optic vesicle is now indented to become a double-walled **optic cup** (Fig. 11.11B,C). Grooves appear on the ventral surface of the optic cup and along the optic stalk forming the **choroidal fissure**. A branch of the ophthalmic artery, the hyaloid artery, passes along the choroidal fissure to supply the lens and the developing retina. Soon the edges of the choroidal fissure fuse, thus enclosing the hyaloid artery and its accompanying vein in a canal. The proximal part of the hyaloid artery persists as the central artery of the retina.

The retina is formed by the two layers of the optic cup, the outer layer forms the pigmented layer of the retina, and the inner or neural layer proliferates to form the rods and cones, and the cell bodies of neurons. The neurons differentiate into bipolar cells, ganglionic cells and neuroglial cells. The axons of the ganglionic cells line the inner surface of the retina and form the optic nerve. At the rim of the optic cup, both layers of the retina give rise to the iris and ciliary body. The neurectoderm overlying the iris forms the connective tissue and the dilator and sphincter pupillae muscles.

The lens is initially a hollow structure. However, soon the posterior cells of the **lens vesicle** elongate to form the lens fibres; these arrange in a laminar pattern to produce a transparent lens (Fig. 11.11C). The mesenchyme around the optic cup condenses to form the layers of the eyeball, the inner vascular choroid and the outer fibrous sclera. The

most anterior part of the cornea becomes transparent (Fig. 11.11D). The spaces that develop in the mesenchyme between the cornea and the lens accumulate secretions from the ciliary body, and enlarge to form the anterior chamber of the eye (Fig. 11.12). A delicate meshwork of fibrous tissue with a gelatinous substance fills the gap between the lens

Clinical box

When the choroidal fissure fails to close during the 6th or 7th week, a cleft appears in the inferior aspect of the iris. If this defect is limited to the iris in the shape of a keyhole, it is known as **coloboma iridis**. It may also extend into the ciliary body and retina.

In **anophthalmos**, the eye is absent and frequently results from failure of the optic vesicle to develop. **Microphthalmia** is a condition in which the eyeball is either too small or almost vestigial. **Congenital detachment of the retina** may occur when the inner and outer layers of the optic cup fail to fuse. In **congenital cataract** the lens is opaque as a result of abnormal development of its fibres. Some congenital cataracts are genetic in origin; others are caused by the rubella virus, or the exposure of the embryo to radiation.

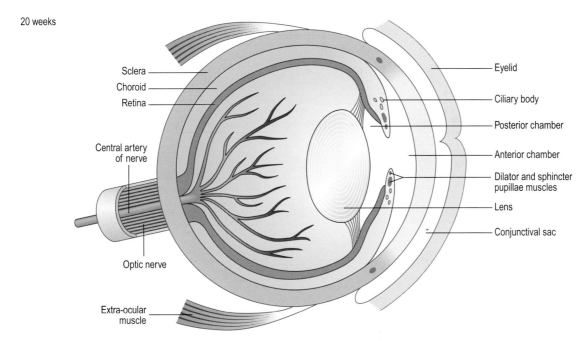

Fig 11.12 **Development of the eye at 20 weeks.**

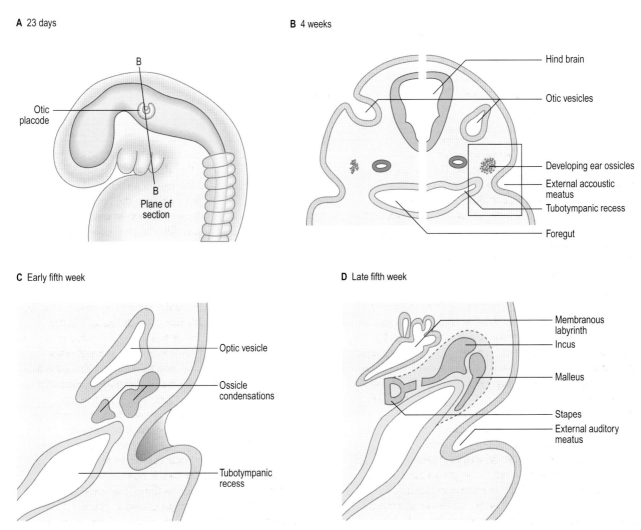

Fig. 11.13 **Development of the ear.** (**A**) embryo at 23 days. (**B**) Coronal section of the embryo. (**C**) Late 5th week. (**D**) Late 5th week.

and the retina, thus forming the vitreous body, which occupies the posterior chamber.

The eyelids develop as folds of ectoderm with mesenchyme between them that grow over the cornea. As the two eyelids grow towards each together, they fuse to enclose a conjunctival sac anterior to the cornea (Fig. 11.12). The inner layer of the ectoderm becomes the conjunctiva and over the iris it fuses with the cornea. The lacrimal glands form as ectodermal buds from the upper part of the conjunctival sac into the surrounding mesenchyme. The eyelids become separated again by 5–7th months in utero.

The ear

The three anatomical subdivisions of the ear have a dual origin. The external and middle ears are derived from the first two pharyngeal arches and from the intervening pharyngeal cleft and pouch. The formation of the external and middle ears is described earlier in this chapter. The inner ear arises from an ectodermal placode that develops at the level of the hindbrain.

The inner ear is first to develop (at about 22 days) as the **otic placode**, close to the hindbrain (Fig. 11.13A). It invaginates as the **otic vesicle** and soon separates from the surface ectoderm (Fig. 11.13B). The optic vesicle enlarges, modifies its shape, forming a dorsal vestibular portion (from which the semicircular canals arise) and a ventral cochlear portion (from which the cochlea arises). A diverticulum arises from the otic vesicle to form the **endolymphatic sac** (Fig. 11.14). The vestibular portion develops two sacs, an expanded larger utricle, and a smaller saccule. Three tubes grow from the utricle to give rise to the semicircular ducts. The lower part of the saccule elongates and spirals as the cochlea. These structures derived from the otic vesicle constitute the membranous labyrinth (Fig. 11.13D). The mesenchyme around the membranous labyrinth becomes the cartilaginous otic capsule; later this is ossified to form the bony labyrinth of the inner ear. The cavities that appear in the otic capsule merge to form a perilymphatic space, which develops the two adult subdivisions, the scala tympani and the scala vestibuli.

> ### Clinical box
> **Congenital deafness** is usually associated with the anomalies of the malleus and incus, which arise from the first pharyngeal arch. A rubella infection during pregnancy may affect the cochlea and its sensory apparatus resulting in **sensorineuronal deafness**.

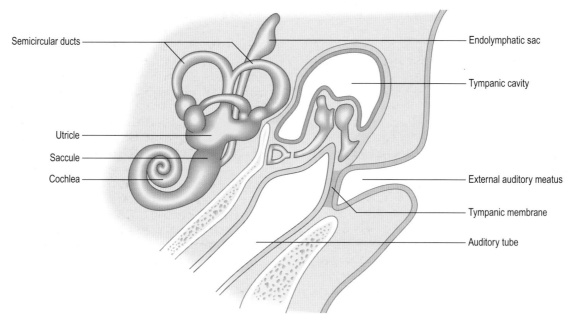

Fig. 11.14 **Development of the membranous labyrinth in a newborn.**

> ### Summary box
> - Five pairs of mesenchymal pharyngeal arches, ectodermal pharyngeal clefts and endodermal pharyngeal pouches develop on either side of the pharyngeal gut.
> - Each pharyngeal arch contains its own cranial nerve, a cartilage and an aortic arch artery.
> - The pharyngeal pouches give rise to the palatine tonsils, the thymus and the parathyroid glands.
> - The tongue develops from a number of swellings on the pharyngeal floor.
> - The thyroid gland arises as a diverticulum from the tongue region.
>
> - The face is formed by the fusion of five facial prominences around the opening of the mouth and the palate from the fusion of an unpaired intermaxillary process and two palatine shelves.
> - The nasal cavity and paranasal sinuses develop from the deepening nasal pits.
> - The eye develops from an outgrowth of the forebrain, an ectodermal placode and the surrounding mesenchyme.
> - The ear begins as an ectodermal placode to form the inner ear. The external and middle ears develop from pharyngeal apparatus.

Glossary

Abembryonic pole – the part of the blastocyst furthest from the inner cell mass

Accessory ribs – non-thoracic ribs, arising from the transverse processes of cervical or lumbar vertebrae

Accessory renal artery – artery(ies) usually supplying the lower pole of the kidney, arising because of the successive vascular supplies as the metanephric kidney 'rises' in its development

Acrania – partial or complete absence of the calvaria or skull bones

Agenesis – failure of an embryonic organ or structure to develop

Alar plates – the dorsal halves of the developing neural tube, separated from the ventral basal plates by the sulcus limitans

Allantois – small outpouching of the endoderm of the yolk sac into the connecting stalk, from which the urachus and thence median umbilical ligament is derived

Amnioblast – a cell derived from the ectoderm which forms the wall of the amniotic cavity, i.e. the amnion

Amnion – the extra-embryonic membrane that surrounds the developing embryo/fetus

Amniotic bands – bands of tissue that detach from the amnion compressing fetal structures, especially limbs

Amniotic cavity – the cavity surrounded by the amnion, filled with amniotic fluid, surrounding the fetus

Amniotic fluid – fluid derived from the amnion and from maternal tissue fluid. It is the fluid lost at the time of the 'breaking of the waters' prior to birth

Ampulla – a flask-like widening of a tube, like the uterine tube

Anal membrane – formed at about 7 weeks, as the cloacal membrane is divided by the urorectal septum

Anchoring villi – the placental villi that attach the chorionic plate to the decidual tissue

Anencephaly – congenital anomaly caused by the failed closure of the anterior neuropore, leading to failure of part or all of the brain to develop

Angiogenic cell cluster – a cluster of mesodermal cells that give rise to blood vessels or the heart tubes

Annular pancreas – a congenital anomaly resulting from splitting of the ventral pancreatic bud such that the two portions migrate and surround the duodenum, thus forming a ring of tissue constricting the gut tube

Anophthalmos – failure of development of the eye

Anterior cardinal vein – vein draining the head region of the fetus, into the common cardinal vein and thus into the sinus venosus

Anterior nares – openings into the nasal cavity on the face

Anterior neuropore – open cranial portion of the neural tube which, after its closure, gives rise to the brain

Aortic arches – the series of initially symmetrical arteries within the pharyngeal arches that arise from the truncus arteriosus to supply structures in the head and neck

Aorticopulmonary septum – spiral partition dividing the ascending aorta and the pulmonary trunk

Atrioventricular canal – the communication between the common atrium and the early ventricle

Atrioventricular groove – the external groove in the heart lying between the atria and the ventricles and in which coronary arteries and the coronary sinus is found

Azygos line veins – one of the pair of initially symmetrical veins (lying in the future trunk) that form the definitive azygos system of veins

Basal plate – the maternal side of the full-term placenta, consisting of the decidua basalis and the syncytiotrophoblast; *alternative meaning* the name given to the ventral thickening of the neural tube

Bicornuate uterus – a mammalian non-primate pattern in which there are two uterine horns, united by a common cervix; this pattern is a relatively common anomaly in humans

Bilaminar embryonic disc – the two adjacent layers of the epiblast/ectoderm and hypoblast/endoderm lying in contact forming the early embryo

Blastocoele – the fluid-filled cavity in the blastocyst

Blastocyst – the hollow sphere of cells derived from the morula consisting of the inner cell mass and the outer trophoblast

Blastomere – component cells of the dividing zygote during cleavage which retains pluripotentiality and forms the morula

Body cavities – serous cavities comprising the pericardial, pleural and peritoneal cavities, all derived form the intra-embryonic coelom

Branchial – resembling the branchia (or 'gills') of fishes and in the human embryo the branchial or pharyngeal arches give rise to structures in the head and neck

Branchial cyst – sometimes as the overgrowing second pharyngeal arch forms a smooth contour to the neck, it encloses a space which is a branchial cyst or a cervical cyst

Branchial fistulae – branchial cysts can sometimes become inflamed, and open via a fistula on to the exterior or the pharynx, anterior to the sternocleidomastoid muscle

Branching morphogenesis – the developmental mechanism responsible for a branching pattern, e.g. of the dividing lung buds

Buccopharyngeal membrane – the place of direct contact between ectoderm and endoderm in the trilaminar embryonic disc which later separates the mouth from the pharynx. It breaks down in week 4 thus establishing communication between the amniotic cavity and the gut tube

Bulboventricular groove – the groove lying between the bulbus cordis and the primitive ventricle in the primitive heart tube

Bulbus cordis – the part of the heart tube that gives rise to the conus cordis (the outflow tract of the ventricles) and the truncus arteriosus which forms the proximal parts of the aorta and the pulmonary trunk

Cardiac loop – the primitive heart tube

Cardiogenic area – the area of unsegmented mesoderm in the trilaminar embryonic disc that gives rise to the heart tube

Cartilaginous plate – the growth plate in a developing long bone

Caudal – the tail end of the embryo

Cephalic – the head end of the embryo

Cephalic flexure – the bend in the cranial part of the developing neural tube in the region of the future midbrain

Cephalocaudal – a term used in relation to the longitudinal (head to tail) folding of the embryo

Cervical flexure – the bend in the developing neural tube between the future medulla and the spinal cord

Cervical rib – an anomalous rib that develops from the transverse process of the 7th cervical vertebra. It may sometimes put pressure on the lower trunk of the brachial plexus or the subclavian artery

Cervical sinus – a space formed by the 2nd, 3rd and 4th pharyngeal clefts enclosed by the overgrowth of the second pharyngeal arch which normally disappears. If it doesn't a cyst may arise

Chordoma – a malignant tumour of the remnants of the notochord

Chorion – the membrane that surrounds the fetus, consisting of trophoblast and extra-embryonic mesoderm

Chorion frondosum – that part of the chorion that is the fetal contribution to the placenta

Chorion laeve – smooth abembryonic wall of the chorion which has lost its villi during the 2nd month. Fuses with the deciduas parietalis and amnion

Chorionic plate – the extra-embryonic mesoderm that lines the cytotrophoblast, thus bordering the chorionic cavity

Chorionic villi – the finger-like protrusions of chorion and trophoblast which contain blood vessels, and are surrounded by maternal blood in the intervillous spaces that allow placental exchange

Choroidal fissure – the groove that forms after the invagination of the optic vesicle and the lens placode on the undersurface of the developing eye

Cleft lip – a congenital anomaly in which there is a split in the upper lip, due to failure of fusion of the components that normally make up the lip. The condition is often associated with a cleft palate

Cleft palate – a congenital anomaly in which the palatal folds that normally fuse in the midline to separate the oral and nasal cavities remain separated, and thus there is free communication between the two cavities

Cloacal fold – seen in the indifferent stage of genital development, the pair of mesenchymal elevations between the genital tubercle and the anal fold, lying around the cloacal membrane

Cloacal membrane – the thin membrane that separates the cloaca from the amniotic cavity; it is divided into an anterior urogenital membrane and a posterior anal membrane by the arrival of the urorectal septum

Cloacal plate – located at the caudal end of the trilaminar embryonic disc, where there is no intervening mesoderm between the ectoderm and endoderm. The plate becomes the cloacal membrane but later breaks down to allow free communication between urogenital structures and the amniotic cavity, and thus the exterior

Coloboma iridis – is a congenital anomaly where the choroid fissure fails to close at the 7th week, and results in a cleft in the iris

Common cardinal veins – the veins in the embryo that receive the anterior and posterior cardinal veins and drain into the sinus venosus

Conceptus – the resulting assembly of tissues at any stage from a fertilized ovum to birth

Congenital cataract – when the lens becomes opaque in utero, usually due to genetic reasons, but can result after maternal rubella infection during pregnancy

Congenital deafness – various structural defects of the middle or inner ear, often caused for genetic reasons, though may follow maternal rubella infection during pregnancy

Congenital detachment of retina – where the outer pigment layer of the retina and the neural layer, initially separated by the intraretinal space, fail to fuse, thus resulting in a detached retina

Conus cordis – the part of the developing heart tube comprising the outflow tracts of the heart, derived from the bulbus cordis, and leading to the truncus arteriosus

Corpus luteum – the remnants of tissue of the Graffian follicle, after the oocyte has left during ovulation, which secretes progesterone

Cotyledons – components of the placenta formed after 4–5 months, divided it into 15–20 structural units (intervillous spaces) by decidual septa

Craniopharyngiomas – usually benign tumours of the pituitary gland derived from the part arising from Rathke's pouch (ectodermal from stomodaeum). They may cause pituitary dysfunction and/or hydrocephalus

Craniosynostosis – premature closure of one or more of the skull sutures

Crista terminalis – the internal ridge in the wall of the right atrium separating the roughened auricular wall from the smooth-walled part derived from the sinus venosus (the sinus venarum)

Cytotrophoblast – the cellular part of the trophoblast, as distinguished from the syncytiotrophoblast

Cytotrophoblast shell – the outer layer of cytotrophoblast that attaches to the decidual plate

Decidual reaction – the process of differentiation of uterine stromal cells following implantation

Decidualization – the process of differentiation of uterine stromal cells following implantation

Decidua basalis – the part of the deciduae that attaches to the cytotrophoblastic shell

Decidua capsularis – the part of the deciduae that covers the abembryonic pole of the implantation site, fusing with the chorion leave and amnion

Decidua parietalis – the part of the deciduae that lines the uterine lumen not involved with implantation

Dermatome – the embryonic structure derived from a somite that contributes, on a segmental basis, to the dermis

Dermomyotome – the embryonic structure derived from a somite that splits into a dermatome and a myotome

Diaphysis – the developing centre of ossification in the shaft of a long bone in endochondral ossification

Diencephalon – the secondary brain vesicle derived from the forebrain that gives rise to the thalamus and hypothalamus

Dizygotic – of two zygotes, term often used in relation to two twins arising from two separate oocytes

Dorsal mesentery – the tissue derived from the lateral plate mesoderm that suspends the gut tube from the dorsal wall of the embryo

Dorsal mesocardium – the membrane that initially suspends the heart tube in the developing pericardial cavity

Dorsal mesogastrium – the part of the dorsal mesentery that suspends the stomach

Dorsal pancreatic bud – the bud of pancreatic tissue derived from foregut endoderm that contributes the larger component to the adult pancreas

Ductus arteriosus – the embryonic vessel that connects the pulmonary trunk to the arch of the aorta, thus providing a means for oxygenated blood to reach the systemic circulation without the need to pass through the lungs

Ductus venosus – the embryonic vessel that lies on the visceral surface of the developing liver and acts as a bypass, thus enabling oxygentated blood in the umbilical vein to gain access to the inferior vena cava (and hence the systemic circulation) without passing through the liver

Dysplasia – abnormal development

Dysplasia of joints – malformation of joints, sometimes caused by pressure of a developing joint against the uterine wall

Ectoderm – the outer germ cell layer that gives rise to the epidermis of the skin, the nervous system and sense organs

Ectodermal placodes – the thickened plate of ectoderm from which sense organs develop

Ectopic – at a site other than the normal one

Embryonic period – from the 3rd to the 8th week of development, during which the embryo is most sensitive to teratogens, and when the organ systems are being formed

Endocardial cushions – mesenchymal structures arising around the atrioventricular canal that divide the latter to form separate channels for the right and left sides of the heart between the atria and ventricles

Endochondral – bone formation from a cartilage model

Endoderm – the inner germ layer from which the lining of the gut tube and its associated glandular structures are derived

Endolymphatic sac – develops as part of the membranous labyrinth of the inner ear

Endometrium – the inner lining of the uterus in which implantation occurs

Epaxial – situated upon or above an axis. The dorsal epimeres of myotomes that give rise to epaxial muscles, the erector spinae muscles

Epiblast – forms the ectoderm germ layer in the early embryo

Epimere – the myotomes give rise to dorsal epimeres which give rise to epaxial muscles, the erector spinae muscles

Epiphyseal – related to the cartilaginous epiphyseal growth plate at which longitudinal growth takes place in a long bone

Epiphysis – the ossification centre of the cartilaginous model of a long bone

Epispadias – congenital anomaly where the urethral opening is on the dorsal surface of the penis and is associated with exstrophy of the urinary bladder

Exocoelomic membrane – the membrane derived from the endoderm that forms the wall of the primitive yolk sac and lines the extra-embryonic coelom

Exstrophy of the urinary bladder – where the mucosa of the urinary bladder is open to the exterior via a defect in the future ventral abdominal wall of the embryo. Always associated with epispadias

Extra-embryonic coelom – the space between the layers of the extra-embryonic mesoderm. Also known as the chorionic cavity, and separates the amnion and yolk sac from the embryo

Extrahepatic biliary atresia – congenital obliteration of parts of the biliary tract potentially causing liver failure if not corrected surgically

Fetal membranes – amnion, chorion, allantois and yolk sac

Fetal period – the period of growth in size of the fetus from week 8 to term

Floating villi – the terminations of chorionic villi that branch off the main stem tertiary villi

Fontanelles – the spaces lying between the flat bones of the fetal skull filled by connective tissue, often referred to as 'soft spots'

Foramen caecum – the depression in the apex of the sulcus terminalis of the tongue that marks the origin of the thyroid gland

Foramen ovale – the hole in the atrial septum in the embryo and fetus allowing oxygenated placental blood in the right side of the heart to pass to the left without going through the pulmonary circulation. Normally this hole closes immediately after birth, forming the fossa ovalis

Forebrain – the most cranial part of the developing brain which gives rise to the cerebral hemispheres and the thalamus and hypothalamus

Fossa ovalis – the depression in the atrial septum marking the site of the closed foramen ovale

Frontonasal prominence – the mesenchymal elevation ventral to the brain vesicles, contributing to the face and constitutes the upper border of the stomodaeum

Gastroschisis – the herniation of the abdominal contents directly through the wall into the amniotic cavity, in which the organs are not invested by amnion or peritoneum

Gastrulation – the process of establishment of the three germ layers

Genital swellings – mesenchymal elevations on either side of the cloacal folds in an indifferent embryo. These become the labia majora in the female or scrotum in the male

Genital tubercle – the forerunner of the glans penis in the male or clitoris in the female

Gonadal ridges – elevations of intermediate mesoderm beneath the coelomic epithelium in the early embryo that give rise to the gonads

Gubernaculum – the band of mesenchyme along which the gonad descends to its definitive adult location

Hepatic diverticulum – the endodermal bud from the foregut that forms the liver

Hepatocardiac channels – venous channels in the fetal liver derived from the two vitelline veins, and draining blood from the ductus venosus to the future inferior vena cava

Hiatal hernia – congenital herniation of the stomach through the oesophageal hiatus in the diaphragm

Hindbrain – the most caudal part of the developing brain that gives rise to the pons and cerebellum, and the medulla oblongata

Horseshoe kidney – a congenital anomaly of the kidney whereby usually the lower poles fuse across the midline giving rise to a horseshoe like appearance

Human chorionic gonadotrophin (HCG) – a hormone produced by the syncytiotrophoblast in sufficient quantities by the end of the 2nd week that it may be detected in urine of pregnant women, thus constituting a test for pregnancy

Hydrocephalus – excessive build up of cerebrospinal fluid leading to enlarged ventricles of the brain, a compressed cerebral cortex and an enlarged skull unless the excess fluid is surgically drained

Hydrocoele – a congenital anomaly of the scrotum in which fluid collects within the tunica vaginalis

Hypaxial – the myotomes give rise to the ventral hypomeres that give rise to hypaxial muscles which include body wall musculature and limb musculature

Hypoblast – gives rise to the endoderm germ layer in the early embryo

Hypobranchial eminence – median swelling in floor of future pharynx, formed from the mesoderm of the second, third and part of the fourth pharyngeal arches. Also known as the copula. Contributes to posterior third of tongue

Hypomere – formed from myotomes and gives rise to lateral and ventral musculature of abdominal and thoracic wall, plus the limb musculature

Hypospadias – incomplete fusion of the urethral folds in the male leading to opening of the penile urethra along its ventral surface

Intermaxillary segment – formed by growth and fusion of parts of the two medial nasal processes and resulting in formation of the philtrum of upper lip and primary palate

Intermediate mesoderm – part of the intra-embryonic mesoderm that gives rise to components of the urogenital system

Intermediate villi – parts of the chorionic villi

Intervillous spaces – blood-filled spaces between the anchoring chorionic villi arising from the trophoblastic lacunae

Intra-embryonic coelom – spaces within the intra-embryonic mesoderm that merge to form the future serous cavities of the trunk

Intra-embryonic mesoderm – the middle layer in the trilaminar disc and the last of the three germ layers of the embryo to form

Intramembranous ossification – ossification process that takes place within mesenchyme (membrane) rather than from a cartilage model

Labioscrotal swellings – arise from the genital swellings that are located on either side of the urethral folds

Lacunae – spaces, hollows or cavities

Lateral lingual swellings – derived from first arch mesoderm which, together with the median tuberculum impar, form the anterior two-thirds of the tongue

Lateral nasal processes – swellings on the outside of the nasal pits that give rise to the lateral side of the nose

Lateral plate mesoderm – most lateral part of intra-embryonic mesoderm that gives rise to the splanchnic and somatic layers: the future visceral and parietal serous membranes of the trunk

Lens placode – thickening of surface ectoderm around forebrain from which the lens vesicle forms

Lens vesicle – invagination of the surface ectoderm from which the lens develops

Levator glandulae thyroideae – lower end of the thyroglossal duct which sometimes gives rise to smooth muscle

Ligamentum arteriosum – fibrosed remnant of the ductus arteriosus connecting the pulmonary trunk and the ascending aorta

Ligamentum teres (hepatis) – fibrosed remnant of the left umbilical vein connecting the umbilicus and the porta hepatis

Ligamentum venosum – fibrosed remnant of the ductus venosus which connects the portal vein to the inferior vena cava

Lobster claw (hand or foot) – abnormal cleft between the second and fourth metacarpal bones and associated soft tissues, with the third bone missing, thus resembling a lobster's claw

Macrostomia – a congenital defect in which there is a large mouth

Mandibular prominence or process – lower part of the first pharyngeal arch that gives rise to lower jaw. Contains Meckel's cartilage which disappears

Mantle layer – part of the developing neural tube closest to the central canal from which grey matter arises

Marginal zone – part of the most peripheral layer of the developing neural tube from which the white matter develops

Maxillary prominence or process – upper part of the first pharyngeal arch that gives rise to the upper jaw

Meckel's cartilage – the cartilaginous part of the lower part of the first pharyngeal arch that disappears, though part of it persists as the sphenomandibular ligament and the malleus and incus

Meckel's diverticulum – the persisting remnant of the vitello-intestinal duct which if inflamed can give rise to symptoms mimicking appendicitis

Medial nasal processes – swellings that form the midline portion of the external nose, and the philtrum of the upper lip

Meningocoele – spina bifida in which the meninges protrude through a dorsal defect in the vertebral canal

Meningomyelocoele – spina bifida in which the meninges and spinal cord tissues protrude through a dorsal defect in the vertebral canal

Mesencephalon – one of the primary brain vesicles that gives rise to the midbrain

Mesenchyme – loose embryonic connective tissue derived from mesoderm or neural crest

Mesoduodenum – the dorsal mesentery associated with the duodenum

Mesonephric duct – duct of the mesonephros which in males partly persists as the ductus deferens, forms the trigone of the urinary bladder, and the ureteric bud of the metanephros

Mesonephros – the primitive kidney that precedes the development of the metanephros, the definitive adult kidney

Metanephric blastema – caudal part of the nephrogenic cord of the intermediate mesoderm into which the ureteric bud grows; the blastema gives rise to the nephrons

Metanephric diverticulum – ureteric buds

Metanephros – the forerunner of the definitive adult kidney that begins in the pelvic region and 'ascends' to its adult lumbar position

Metencephalon – the secondary brain vesicle that gives rise to the pons and cerebellum, arising from the rhombencephalon

Microcephaly – congenital defect in which the brain fails to develop and the head is small

Microphthalmia – a small eyeball

Microstomia – congenital defect in which there is a small mouth

Monozygotic – term related to identical twins in which a single ovum gives rise to two individuals

Morula – the result of the mitotic divisions of the zygoyte prior to the formation of the blastocyst

Muscular dystrophy – congenital myopathy leading to muscle degeneration and weakness

Myelencephalon – the secondary brain vesicle that gives rise to the medulla, arising from the rhombencephalon

Myoblast – precursor cells of muscle, derived from intra-embryonic mesoderm

Myotome – part of a somite that gives rise to somatic muscle

Nasal pits – openings derived from the nasal placodes

Nasal placodes – invaginations from the surface ectoderm giving rise to nasal pits

Nasal sacs – deepenings of the nasal pits forming the nasal cavities

Nasolacrimal groove – the deep furrow separating the medial and lateral nasal prominences, and from which the nasolacrimal duct forms

Nephric vesicle – the early tubule into which the glomeruli invaginate, and which links up with the duct system of the developing kidney

Nephrogenic cord – intermediate mesoderm tissue that gives rise to pro-, meso- and metanephric tissues

Neural crest – apical portion of the neural groove, budding off prior to formation of the neural tube. Gives rise to a wide range of structures including components of the peripheral and autonomic nervous system

Neural crest cells – neuroectodermal cells forming the neural crest

Neural folds – edges of the neural groove, the apical edges of which meet in the midline to form the neural tube

Neural groove – the midline furrow in surface ectoderm which differentiates to form the neural tube

Neural plate – the slipper-shaped enlargement of the surface ectoderm which rounds up, initially forming the neural groove and then the neural tube

Neural tube – the forerunner of the brain and spinal cord

Neuroblasts – cells of the mantle zone of the developing neural tube that give rise to neurons

Neurocranium – the skull, including its vault and base

Neuroectoderm – the specialized part of the surface ectoderm that gives rise to the neural tube and associated nervous structures

Neuroepithelial cells – cells of the neuroepithelial layer

Neuroepithelial layer – cells that give rise to the rest of the wall of the neural tube, and itself differentiates into the ependymal cells lining the tube

Neurulation – the process of neural tube formation

Notochord – the midline structure that forms a midline axis for the embryo, and from which the intervertebral discs are formed

Notochordal plate – cells arising from the primitive pit to form the cylinder which becomes the notochord

Oblique facial cleft – result from the failure of the maxillary prominence to fuse with its partner lateral nasal prominence

Occipital myotomes – myotomes in the occipital region of the embryo, some of which give rise to the musculature of the tongue

Oesophageal atresia – failure of the oesophagus to develop

Oesophageal hernia – a form of diaphragmatic hernia in which upper parts of the stomach are located above the diaphragm because of congenital shortness of the oesophagus, and hence there may be a constriction in the stomach

Omphalocele – herniation of abdominal contents through the umbilical ring, covered by amnion

Optic cup – double-walled invagination of the optic vesicle

Optic stalk – the stalk-like hollow evagination of part of the forebrain which produces the cup-like retina into which the lens vesicle fits

Oronasal membrane – separates the oral cavity from the future nasal cavity before the membrane breaks down

Ostium primum – the first opening in the developing atrial septum that disappears as the septum primum reaches the endocardial cushion

Ostium secundum – second foramen to form in the upper part of the septum primum which forms the foramen ovale of the atrial septum

Otic placode – thickening of ectoderm on each side of the hindbrain from which the otic vesicle forms

Otic vesicle – invagination of the otic placode from which the inner ear develops

Ovum – fertilized secondary oocyte

Paired heart tubes – endocardial tubes formed from mesenchymal angiogenic cell clusters that fuse to form a single heart tube after folding of the embryo

Paramesonephric ducts – paired ducts derived from the coelomic epithelium. Fuse in the midline to form the uterus and uterine tubes

Paraxial mesoderm – mesodermal cells close to the midline between the ectoderm and the endoderm, from which somites arise

Parietal – of the body walls (paries = wall, Latin)

Pelvic kidney – congenital condition in which the developing kidney does not undergo 'ascent' to achieve its adult position and remains in the pelvis

Pericardioperitoneal canals – part of the intra-embryonic coelom from which the pleural cavities develop

Pharyngeal arches – 5/6 paired mesodermal structures in the developing pharyngeal wall from which certain components of the head and neck are derived

Physiological umbilical hernia – protrusion of part of the developing intestinal loop into the umbilicus during elongation and rotation of the midgut

Placenta previa – a placenta that develops over the internal os of the uterus

Placental septa – partitions of the placenta formed by decidual tissue thus resulting in 15–20 cotyledons (compartments in the placenta)

Pleuropericardial folds – membranes that separate the pericardial cavity from the pleural cavities

Pleuroperitoneal membranes – folds that separate the future pleural from the peritoneal cavities

Pluripotential – potential of developing in more than one way, or a number of fixed points of differentiation

Polydactyly – congenital condition in which additional digits on hands or feet develop

Polyhdramnios – an excess of amniotic fluid possibly resulting from an inability of the fetus to swallow as a consequence of oesophageal atresia

Posterior neuropore – caudal opening in the neural tube which closes on the 27th day

Primary brain vesicles – three dilatations at the cranial end of the neural tube that give rise to the secondary brain vesicles and thence the cerebrum, cerebellum and brain stem

Primary chorionic villi – trophoblastic projections in the developing placenta. Gaseous exchange will occur after the appearance of a mesenchymal core (secondary villi) in which blood vessels develop (tertiary villi)

Primary yolk sac – formed by the lining of the endoderm cells which migrate around the lower portion of the blastocyst cavity

Primitive cloaca – endoderm-derived cavity at the terminal part of the hindgut which forms the rectum and upper anal canal, and the urinary bladder

Primitive node – rim of ectoderm at the cranial end of the primitive streak giving rise to the notochord

Primitive pit – a depression located around the primitive node

Primitive sex cords – structures in the presumptive gonads that come to be occupied by the primordial germ cells that migrate from the yolk sac

Primitive streak – a linear midline structure derived from epiblast/ectoderm whose migrating cells form the mesoderm germ layer

Primitive urogenital sinus – the ventral component resulting from the partitioning of the cloaca comprising the urinary bladder and urethra

Primordia – the beginning formations of a structure

Primordial germ cells – cells that migrate from the wall of the yolk sac to occupy the sex cords in the gonads and give rise to either oogonia or spermatogonia

Probe patency of the foramen ovale – a common developmental anomaly in which there is incomplete sealing of the foramen ovale, such that it is possible to pass a probe from one atrial chamber to the other

Processus vaginalis – the part of the peritoneal cavity that precedes the testis through the inguinal canal, and into which the testis invaginates. Later in development the processus becomes the tunica vaginalis

Prochordal plate – an area at the cranial end of the embryonic disc where there is contact between the ectoderm and the endoderm, and no intervening mesoderm. The forerunner of the buccopharyngeal membrane

Proctodaeum – the ectodermal depression from the surface ectoderm that forms the lower part of the anal canal

Pronephros – first primitive kidney formation that disappears completely, superseded by the mesonephros and thence the metanephros

Prosencephalon – primary brain vesicle from which the telencephalon and diencephalon form

Pulmonary hypoplasia – underdevelopment of the lung in which there is a reduced number of air sacs or alveoli

Rachischisis – spina bifida in which neural fold tissue remains open on the dorsal surface of the back

Rathke's pouch – an ectodermal outpocketing of the stomodeum (the ectodermal part of the lining of the oral cavity) from which the anterior lobe of the pituitary develops

Respiratory distress syndrome – condition in which the alveoli collapse due to lack of surfactant production by the type II alveolar epithelial cells

Respiratory diverticulum – outpouching of the foregut endoderm that gives rise to the epithelial lining and glands of the trachea and bronchial tree

Rhombencephalon – most caudal of the three primary cerebral vesicles that gives rise to the metencephalon (pons and cerebellum) and the myelencephalon (medulla)

Rostral – relating to the beak, or in humans the nose; term used to define a position at the head end of the embryo

Scaphocephaly – an abnormally long and narrow skull due to premature closing of the sagittal suture, with centres of ossification in the suture line

Sclerotome – derived from the somite and giving rise to connective tissue surrounding the neural tube and notochord to form the vertebrae

Secondary chorionic villi – placental villi whose core contains mesenchymal tissue

Secondary yolk sac – derived from the overgrowth of endodermal cells around the wall of the primary yolk sac

Sensorineuronal deafness – a hearing loss due to a lesion in the cochlea or in the auditory nerve or its pathway to the brain, sometimes caused by maternal rubella infection at the time of pregnancy

Septum primum – a sickle-shaped growth in the roof of the common atrium that extends towards the endocardial cushions leaving the opening of the foramen primum

Septum secundum – a second crescent-shaped fold forming part of the developing atrial septum, after the appearance of the septum primum. Together the two septa form the atrial septum

Septum transversum – unsegmented mesoderm that develops initially cranial to the prochordal plate, and gives rise to part of the diaphragm, the fibrous pericardium, and connective tissues of the liver. It migrates from its original position in the cervical region of the embryo to its adult position

Sinus venarum – the smooth-walled part of the developing right atrium

Sinus venosus – the venous channel that drains blood into the heart from the embryo and the placenta. Initially, it is a symmetrical structure having two horns, but with time it loses its symmetry, and the numbers of veins that drain into it. In the adult only the coronary sinus, the smooth part of the right atrium, and the proximal portion of the inferior vena cava persist

Sinuvaginal bulbs – endodermal swellings from the posterior wall of the urogenital sinus forming the lower part of the vagina

Somatic mesoderm – derived from the lateral plate mesoderm and forming the serous membrane associated with the body wall

Somatopleure – somatic lateral plate mesoderm

Somites – most medial segmented components differentiated from the paraxial mesoderm and giving rise to muscle of the trunk and limbs, most of the axial skeleton and part of the dermis

Spina bifida cystica – a neural tube defect in which the neural tube and/or surrounding membranes protrudes through a deficient vertebral arch posteriorly forming a cyst-like structure and resulting in neurological deficits

Spina bifida occulta – a less severe form of spinal bifida in which the neural tube tissue remains in its normal location, but with a deficient posterior vertebral arch. The defect is often marked by an overlying patch of hairy skin

Splanchnic mesoderm – lateral plate mesoderm that gives rise to the serous membranes covering viscera (splanchnic = pertaining to organs)

Splanchnopleure – splanchnic lateral plate mesoderm

Sternal bars – bars of cartilage (sternebrae) from which the sternum develops

Stomodaeum – ectodermal invagination forming part of the oral cavity, and bordering with the endodermal-lined portion which is the pharynx

Subcardinal – term used in relation to one of the longitudinal veins draining the body of the embryo that is incorporated into the inferior vena cava

Sulcus limitans – the longitudinal groove that separates the alar and basal plates of the parts of the neural tube that give rise to the derivatives of the diencephalon (thalamus and hypothalamus), brain stem and spinal cord

Sulcus terminalis – the groove on the exterior of the heart that marks the crista terminalis, demarcating the smooth-walled from the roughened parts of the right atrium

Supracardinal – term used in relation to one of the longitudinal veins draining the body of the embryo that becomes part of the azygos system

Surfactant – the phospholipid substance produced by type II alveolar cells that reduces surface tension at the air:alveolar interface and thus facilitates respiration

Syncytiotrophoblast – the outer part of the trophoblast that invades the endometrium and which contributes to the formation of the placenta

Telencephalon – one of the pair of secondary cerebral vesicles from the forebrain that gives rise to the cerebral hemispheres

Teratogen – an agent that can cause a birth defect

Tertiary villi – a chorionic villus that has blood vessels in its core

Thyroglossal duct – duct leading from the apex of the sulcus terminalis of the tongue at the foramen caecum to the developing thyroid gland. Sometime this duct persists in part of its course giving rise to ectopic thyroid tissue

Thyroglossal fistula – an abnormal connection of the thyroglossal duct to the exterior

Thyroid diverticulum – the endodermal bud of tissue migrating from the foramen caecum to form the thyroid gland

Tracheo-oesophagal fistula – an abnormal communication between the developing oesophagus and trachea

Truncoconal swellings – develop in the conus cordis and the truncus arteriosus to form the aortico-pulmonary septum which divides the ascending aorta and the pulmonary trunk

Tuberculum impar – midline swelling in the floor of the pharynx derived from the first pharyngeal arch mesoderm and contributes to the anterior two-thirds of the tongue

Tubotympanic recess – first pharyngeal pouch that further develops as the auditory tube

Ultimobranchial body – derived from the lower part of the fourth (sometimes considered to be the fifth) pharyngeal pouch from which the parafollicular or 'C' cells of the thyroid gland develop

Umbilical arteries – blood vessels bringing deoxygenated blood to the placenta from the fetus

Umbilical cord – the composite of structures linking the fetus with the placenta. Contains the yolk sac remnants, vitelline duct remnants, umbilical vessels and is covered by amnion

Umbilical veins – blood vessels bringing oxygentated blood to the fetus from the placenta. Only the left umbilical vein persists and after birth it becomes the ligamentum teres of the liver

Urachus – the fibrous cord that connects the urinary bladder to the umbilicus. It arises from the allantois; if this remains patent urachal sinuses, cysts or fistulae may result

Uterovaginal canal – fused paramesonephric ducts that becomes the uterus and the upper part of the vagina

Ureteric bud – develops from the caudal end of the mesonephric duct growing into the nephrogenic cord with which it forms the metanephros

Urethral folds – arise from the cloacal folds forming the labia minora in females and the shaft of the penis in males

Urogenital membrane – the anterior half of the cloacal membrane that covers the urogenital openings, and later breaks down

Urogenital ridge – derived from the intermediate mesoderm bulging into the coelomic cavity from which kidneys, ureters and parts of the reproductive system develop

Urogenital sinus – anterior division of the cloaca giving rise to the urinary bladder and the urethra

Urorectal septum – mesodermal tissue that partitions the cloaca into a ventral urogenital sinus and a dorsal anorectal canal

Uteroplacental circulation – the circulation in which the transport of substances between the maternal and fetal blood occurs across the walls of the chorionic villi

Ventral mesentery – the mesentery associated with the foregut derived from the septum transversum

Ventral pancreatic bud – the smaller of the two buds of endodermal tissue from the foregut that gives rise to part of the head and the uncinate process of the pancreas

Visceral – organ or viscus, thus visceral relating to an organ

Viscerocranium – bones that give rise to the face mainly derived from the first two pharyngeal arches

Vitelline duct – the connection between the yolk sac and the midgut. Sometimes a proximal portion of it persists as Meckel's diverticulum

Vitelline veins – veins draining the yolk sac, some of which become the drainage of the gut, as branches of the hepatic portal vein

Vitello-intestinal duct – vitelline duct

Volvulus – a twisting of the intestines with a risk of cutting off blood supply

Zona pellucida – the thick membrane that surrounds an oocyte

Index